# Illuminating PHYSICAL Experience

To Order Additional Copies Call
Toll-free number: 1-877-328-1744
www.kornax.com

Dr. Marcy Foley Davidsson
William L. Shaffer
Kent Davidsson

Edited by Donald Johnson

*Illuminating Physical Experience*



Printed at Central Plains Book Manufacturing, Kansas
Cover Photo Copyright by Ralph A. Clevenger/CORBIS
Cover Design by Bob Schram, Bookends

Davidsson, Marcy Foley.
Illuminating PHYSICAL experience / Marcy Foley Davidsson, William L. Shaffer, Kent Davidsson ; edited by Donald Johnson. -- 1st ed.
p. cm.
ISBN: 0-9631452-4-X

1. Holistic medicine. 2. Mental healing. 3. Mind and body. 4. Health--Religious aspects. 5. Self-actualization (Psychology) 6. Alternative medicine. I. Shaffer, William L. II. Davidsson, Kent. III. Johnson, Donald. IV. Title

R733.D38 2000 615.5
QBI00-532

# Table of Contents

## Chapter 1
## What it Means to Heal



## Chapter 2
## Impediments to Healing



## Chapter 3
## Emotional Ownership

## Chapter 4
## Body Symbology & Taking Personal Responsibility

## Chapter 5
## The Creation of Our Lives

## Appendix I
## Chakras



## Appendix II
## Therapies for Self-Healing



## Epilogue

# Chapter 1
# What It Means to Heal

## Why We Have Disease, Pain & Suffering

This is not a typical book about healing. It is a book about awakening your consciousness by recognizing and owning aspects of yourself that you have long forgotten. It is a book about remembering and understanding . . . understanding leading to wisdom . . . and applied wisdom leading to enlightenment. Most importantly, this book is about taking responsibility for all that you create by engaging in emotional ownership.

We cannot heal what we don't see, so our Creator has given us each other and a three-dimensional planet. We see ourselves in each other as perfect mirrors. Everything on the third dimensional plane is here to mirror our patterns and our consciousness.

For example, our consciousness is symbolized through our bodies and material possessions. We need these things to function in third-dimensional existence. However, these items also give us clues about our state of consciousness. Since Earth is a planet where most of us reject our ability to communicate telepathically, we communicate through spoken or written communication and through our bodies. Many incarnate souls on this planet aren't even aware that there is more to us than our physical bodies.

In such a world, how is God to show us things about ourselves to help us along our path and teach us? One way to get our attention is through changes in the physical body. In the beginning we may ignore a small ache or pain, some small muscle twitch, or a loss of body function. However, the Universe in It's infinite love and compassion will keep intensifying this signal until we finally pay attention. If we still don't, the aches and pains will get even more severe until we do pay attention.

It is interesting to note people's reactions to this amplification technique. Some get angry at God for turning up the signal so we can "hear" it. Others feel they are being punished by God. It is all a matter of one's picture of reality, which includes how souls perceive their Creator, the Universe, the Cosmos, or whatever you choose to call this Force that permeates all existence. Some call this All That Is, the Life Force, or just Life. It doesn't matter. What does matter is *your relationship* to this energy.

How you view the Creative Energies is a wonderful place to start with your journey into yourself. Some people see God as a fatherly figure wearing a white robe, sitting on a cloud while the angels play their harps and flutes. Some see God as an external force that makes it all happen here on Earth. Some see everything as a manifestation of the Universal Creative Force. Some people believe that we get sick when we "offend" God, and all we have to do is submit to God again and *voilá* — healing is instantaneous! Some people think they just have to find the "right" medicines or healer and then all will be well again.

Some feel that disease, pain and suffering are punishments from God. Some Christians believe that because they have the Holy Spirit, they should be exempt from experiences of discomfort, pain or disease. Other people feel that doing enough "good" deeds will save them from their perceived punishments of God.

Some people say faith is the only solution. All we have to do is say our prayers and trust that God will heal us. When they see someone who is very ill, they may point fingers and judge that person, saying "you lack faith."

Listen! There is no separation between you and God. You are God and God is you. The Creator cannot be separate from the Creation. God would not punish you because God would not punish Itself. Love is not something that we "earn" once we are good enough, have said enough prayers, affirmations, or done enough good deeds. Love isn't something that can be given to or taken away from you. Love isn't something you can *not* be, because you *are* love. Love is who you are.

However, sometimes we can *feel* there's an absence of love in us. We can *feel* unlovable. We can *feel* incapable. We can *feel* unappreciated. We can *feel* like we are stupid. Even though we experience these feelings or perceptions (albeit misperceptions), they are not the Truth. When we experience these issues, illness often happens in our bodies in some form or another. This is one way the Creator can help us in seeing our misperceptions. All of us have issues, patterns and ways of denying True Reality. Most of these involve judging, criticizing and rejecting ourselves until we feel unlovable, incapable or unacceptable.

Our emotional bodies are true gifts from God because they give us "feelers" or "probes" with which to experience life. Many of us still see our emotions as the enemy — something to be eradicated, squelched, gotten rid of, repressed or denied. However, it is through our emotional bodies that we can give a passionate response to our day-to-day experiences. Unfortunately, many people do not value feeling and *owning* their emotions. Many people are so congested, confused and "tired of it all" that they blame others for how they themselves feel.

Projection can sometimes be a very useful tool. We all do it. We project something which is inside of us onto someone else so that we can see it, own it and heal it. Energy of any kind cannot be "gotten rid of." Energy can be transformed, changed, and directed differently. However, energy cannot be ignored or discarded. Energy that is present is there for a reason. Look and see what is in your body, what is in your environment, and who are the people with whom you have relationships.

In order to be healed, one needs to discern energies. Why are certain energies present? Why are we drawn to particular healers, remedies and pathways? All of these have something to teach us. There are no accidents, no mistakes, no victims.

Everyone is always in a process of restoring wholeness and integrity within the body. Remember, what is manifested in the physical is *always* a mirror or reflection of something happening in one of our subtle bodies, (or on some level of our consciousness) which vibrates at a higher frequency of energy.

If you want to know what ideas you have about men, simply look at what kind of men you have in your life.[1] Do you have men who abuse you, criticize you, seek to control you and lash out at you? Then this is your picture of masculine energies. Granted, it is a distorted picture which contains images of *imbalanced masculine energies* . . . but then most people don't know the difference between balanced and

[1] We will thoroughly discuss the difference between "a male" and "masculine energies" in this book. They are not synonymous. However, this is just used as an example because we use men to symbolize masculine energies for us.

imbalanced masculine energies. Most people have never seen true masculine or feminine energies.

Do you want to know your ideas about God the Father? Then look and see what kind of an earthly father you have created. Does he tell you that you have to earn his love by doing enough good things in order to please him? Does he punish you when you don't follow his wishes? Can you really *feel* his love for you?

What ideas do you have about relationships? Why do you keep having relationships that turn out to bring up the same issues and patterns in you even though you keep changing partners? If you want your relationships and external reality to be different, it is necessary for you to re-evaluate your internal beliefs and own your internal emotions. These and other topics we will explore in this book. Most importantly, we will show you *how* to take emotional ownership and responsibility for your life.

Some people feel that if they just eat the right diet and take the right supplements, then they can be free of all disease. This is especially true in people who don't wish to engage in emotional ownership. They simply look to third-dimensional reasons for things in this *and only this* lifetime, and that's all there is — so they think.

There is no one cause for disease or for any of the other challenges we all face as humans on this planet. Yes, there are some generalities which we will discuss in Chapter Four on "Body Symbology." However, no one but you knows the unique set of characteristics that are a compilation of the thousands of lifetimes you have lived.

Some people wonder why "Sally Smith" took "xyz" supplements and cleared her disease, but when "Frances" (who had the same physical symptoms as Sally) came along and took those very same supplements, it didn't do a thing for her. This is because Sally had already done extensive emotional ownership work and accepted responsibility for what she had created, so her Higher Self allowed her to discover a physical substance that would make the difference. She had already cleared up the problem at the level of the *Source.*

The difference is that Frances doesn't believe that the mind or the emotions have anything to do with physical disease, and she refuses to consider this possibility. So her Higher Self will not allow her to "find" the solution until she takes responsibility for her actions. We have given you many tools in this book to go deep within yourself and discover all the judgments and emotions you have hidden inside of you, which have been preventing you from healing yourself.

One of the most important films to come out of Hollywood in recent years is *What Dreams May Come.* This film chronicles the journey of a doctor, portrayed by Robin Williams, who dies in a car accident several years after his two children were also killed in a car accident. Then, after the doctor's death, his wife commits suicide. The film illustrates what discarnate souls may experience after death, determined by a soul's belief systems, expectations and emotions.

Many souls believe that if they see Jesus after death (or in a near-death experience), this confirms that Jesus is indeed the Savior and Christianity is the correct religion. What is imperative to understand here is that life does not validate or confirm anything. It merely reflects. If you look in the mirror and see a physically beautiful (or ugly) person, the mirror is not proving or confirming that you are beautiful or ugly. A mirror simply reflects. What is beautiful or ugly is determined by your choice to perceive or judge in a particular way.

Physical life is a mirror. It's purpose is not to justify, prove or validate anything. Life reflects. Nothing is true or not true simply by what happens or by what is observed. It is our thoughts, feelings, beliefs, fears and expectations that manufacture what we choose to accept or deny, validate or invalidate.

Your life experience doesn't prove or disprove anything. It reflects your thoughts, feelings, beliefs and expectations. You then must determine what to do with that information and experience. *What Dreams May Come* is a powerful film to illustrate this truth and help individuals look at themselves and their lives in a whole new perspective. We highly recommend this film to assist you on your life's path and as an illustration of what we wish to convey in this book.

The following pages explore the various aspects which are within us, mostly those aspects which have been repressed or denied expression and ownership. This has been going on for thousands of lifetimes. *Denial is no longer appropriate if we are to evolve beyond the third dimension.* If we don't address our previously denied energies, we will be sent to another third-dimensional planet until we "get it," or until we take ownership and reclaim those lost aspects of ourselves, which we refer to in this book as our lost will.

This book is meant to stimulate you, to bring you into full experience and acceptance of your emotions, patterns and issues. You may feel hurt, angry or resentful. You may want to throw this book against the wall in a fit of rage. What is appropriate is that you honestly feel that which comes forth from within you. Since you drew this book to you, it means you are ready for this information *on some level*, and you are ready to make some powerful changes in your life.

There was a reason that you chose the country of your birth and also the country where you currently reside if it is different from your country of origin. There was a reason you chose your sex and sexual preference, your religion, lack of religion, your race, your parents (including your genetics) and siblings. The information which follows will give you clues so that you can discern why you made the choices that you made. The important points are to honor, respect, love, own, and take full responsibility for your choices. As you do so, you will accelerate your healing process.

# Chapter 2
# Impediments to Healing

## Necessity of Third Dimensional Existence

Before third-dimensional existence we existed as group energy/group consciousness. There was a sense of comfort, safety and belonging in this group unity. However, there was a blockage to Cosmic Evolution because we identified ourselves according to our placement in this group dynamic. An identification as an individual consciousness was always lacking. This is what lead to the necessity of third-dimensional existence. We were all part of a group existence. Our next choice was to experience ourselves fully as individuals in order to encompass our being on all levels and to recognize our addicted attachment to group connection.

From the onset of third-dimensional incarnation, most human souls immediately went into deep panic and terror. The memory of oneness resulted in most souls perceiving individuality in physical bodies as separation from the group. We then judged the separation as rejection and abandonment by the original group totality. That's why most of us, from our very first incarnation in the third dimension, have focused on getting out of physical existence as fast as possible. This only further stimulated our panic, terror and isolation, as well as the expectation that these painful emotions would forever go on until we could find some way to get back "home."

There are still enormous reservoirs of this original panic, fear, self-judgment and negative expectation deeply suppressed in the subconscious of most incarnate souls. Rather than allowing ourselves to meet this energy and feel these original emotions, we have tried to escape by finding purpose, worthiness, meaning and self-value in external missions. We hoped some external God would then take pity on us and say, "You've done well. You can come home now."

There is no exclusively external God. We have no home outside of us. Although we do experience many forms and levels of service to each other, these are not the *primary mission* but rather the *natural expression* of our true primary mission: to explore, feel and be ourselves fully and completely.

The lack of awareness of this truth or the lack of trust in this truth continues to propel souls to seek external validation through serving others. What we do is always a mere projection of our internal being. We are all here to help each other, but only by being ourselves as totally as possible. The Universe never has and never will ask us to deny ourselves love, joy, happiness, prosperity, relationship, home or anything else. The Universe asks only that we see and own the true deepest motivation behind our thoughts, emotions, reactions, beliefs and expectations.

Vows of denial, for example, are simply projections of an untrusting, fearful human consciousness trying to save itself from what it assumes is punishment for not being good enough. We were not sent into physical existence out of any judgment or punishment. We did nothing wrong. We made no mistakes. We simply chose third-dimensional experience because we lacked emotional feeling and experience of ourselves. This was preventing our natural evolution as part of the Cosmos.

Our vows are projections of what we are afraid to feel, own or recognize within us. We can make all the affirmations we want. We can send Light anywhere our hearts desire, but it will not create true clearing and healing until there is full emotional ownership within us.

It is important to neither judge any emotions, nor to be afraid to feel fear or insecurity. For most of us, terror was the very first emotion we ever experienced. This still requires healing. So long as we are afraid to feel terror, we are bound to physical existence. When we can feel fear and not be afraid of feeling the fear, we have begun the process of healing this deep emotional denial.

Souls have tried to convince themselves that if they do enough or believe enough, they will be saved. Many souls even manipulate religion to make God into a limited projection of human understanding. This creates safety nets and escape routes to avoid dealing with total self-creative responsibility and ownership. The Universe does not care what we do or believe. We do not evolve by knowing anything, believing anything, understanding anything, or even doing anything. We evolve by feeling and being one hundred per cent what we create and experience in each moment.

Allow yourself to honor and feel your emotions without judging them or needing to get rid of them. Simply feel them for what they are trying to show you about yourself. Also remember that although everything you feel is real, not everything you feel is necessarily true. For example, if you feel unworthy of love, this is a real feeling but it is not true. You must allow yourself to feel whatever emotion is there. Then choose whether or not it is *your* truth. In any given moment, stop and ask yourself these three important questions:

*What am I feeling in this moment?*
*What does this feeling tell me about myself?*
*What do I choose to do with this?*

If you answer these three simple questions fully and honestly, they will lead you to the deepest learning, the deepest self-recognition, the deepest ownership of who you are and who you choose to be. You will invoke a change in your life by rescinding the old vows, beliefs and expectations that have caused you pain and limited your joy.

## Vows: We'll Have "NUN" of That!

Across the centuries, our families, governments, churches and spiritual groups have asked us to take vows of commitment to service, growth, love or spiritual development. We have willingly taken on these vows in our lack of self-trust and self-value, hoping these rituals would provide the acceptance, validity, identity and value we were unwilling to give to ourselves. Certainly, there has been much genuine motivation and desire to serve, improve, grow and be the best we could for others. At the same time, vows and the rituals attached to them were all too often created by churches or governments out of a distrustful need to dominate and control others. We gave into them because they reflected our lack of trust and honoring within ourselves.

It is very useful to remember the vows that we made in this or other life experiences so that we can rescind them. Vows remain in place in the very cells of our bodies until they are consciously rescinded.

Some of us wonder why we don't have enough money, even though we work on our affirmations and visualizations. Many of us wonder why our relationships and sex lives aren't as fulfilling as we wish they were. Many of us wonder why we give in or listen to outside authority figures when we really want to go within and listen to our own reality. Most of all, we wonder why we have such low self-esteem. All of these things are often due to old vows that now need to be rescinded and replaced with an energy of self-sovereignty.

Of all the vows we could rescind, the most urgent are the ones we made in lifetimes as monks or nuns. These were vows of poverty, chastity, obedience and humility. For the past two thousand years, whenever we wanted to live a life devoted to spiritual aspirations, the only option available to us was usually within religious structures. The first step now is to recognize and remember that we took these vows. The second step is to understand *why* we took these vows and then to discover the energy underneath these vows that still holds them in place. The third step is letting that vow go.

Rescinding a vow begins by saying something like the following (Choose words that are meaningful and powerful for you):

> *"I formally rescind any and all vows in the areas of poverty, chastity, obedience and humility. I ask all the energies that still support or maintain these vows to now be transmuted into pure Light. I command all cellular memory of these vows in my body to be dissolved now and forever. I now call forth new energies of financial abundance, sexual satisfaction, adherence to my own inner truth and the joy of true self-love. I recognize, accept and honor the lessons I chose in these past lifetimes. Now I am truly and fully finished and set free of all vows of self-denial."*

One of the most difficult lessons for human souls to learn is that merely understanding something or invoking something will not in itself cause the result we seek. *It is of the utmost importance to re-connect to the emotional energy that caused us to choose these self-limitations in the first place.* Only by allowing ourselves to reconnect with the original emotional patterns can we then understand why we originally chose the vows.

These emotional patterns are often based on a sense of purposelessness that requires some external mission. For example, the most common question asked during an Akashic reading is, "What is my mission in life?" The expectation is always about something *external* involving other people. However, your true mission in life is just to be yourself one hundred per cent. This means not only understanding and knowing but also *feeling* who you create yourself to be. Most souls do not trust this inner truth.

Let us get this straight right now: There is no such thing as good or bad karma. There is no such thing as karmic reward or karmic punishment, and the Universe never judges or punishes us out of any sense of blame or fault. These concepts are illusions that exist solely in the mind of a guilt-ridden humanity.

Things do not happen to us because of what we have done in the past. We are not murdered because we have murdered. We are not robbed because we have robbed. We create our experiences ourselves, based on unresolved emotional issues. We are robbed, murdered or whatever only because we think we deserve to be punished. Karma is simply energy balancing itself. There is nothing moralistic, judgmental, rewarding or punishing in it. It is our belief systems, our expectations, our fears and all the emotional reactions that come from these aspects of us that determine what experiences we choose for ourselves.

Many of us are also trapped in the belief that we cannot evolve without suffering — that suffering is growth. We worship martyrdom, hoping that if we suffer enough, someone or something outside of us will save us. This has been distorted so much that many of us choose to believe that a God-like being incarnated to suffer for us.

No suffering is needed to achieve healing and growth. Pain is not a feeling. It is resistance to feeling. Suffering and pain are created in direct proportion to one's fearful self-denial or to the denial of that denial. It is true that we can heal and grow from suffering experiences because they can teach us things about how and what we resist, but *this method of learning is not a requirement.* It is not necessary. It is not expected, demanded or even preferred by the Universe.

Still, many hold on to vows of service and growth based on a need to suffer in order to purify themselves. This need exists only in their guilty minds. Pain, suffering or loss of any kind in one's life is not a judgment or punishment.

For example, if we lose our home and all our possessions in a tornado, this is not some capricious external God throwing an experience at us so that we will suffer and grow from it. Nor is it a punishment for some negative past deed. But if we base our worth on what we have, we may have chosen to experience losing the external possessions to show us the untruth of that belief. Some may have chosen such an experience because of some past vow to suffer. Others may have used the opportunity of the tornado because they carry a subconscious wish to punish themselves out of guilt over actions, thoughts or feelings they have, or have had in the past. Whatever the reason is for choosing a traumatic experience of any kind, it always presents us with two choices. Either we take responsibility for having manifested the situation at hand and embrace with ownership the emotions that the experience brings to the surface in us. Or we choose to feel victimized and even further dis-own those emotions and the power to manifest our reality.

Nothing we choose is ever "carved in stone." We are not forever bound to any choices we make. As our own creative masters, we can un-choose and re-choose to our heart's content. To ask yourself, "What should I do?" and then feel guilty if you want to do something else is just like committing yourself to one of those old vows. Take the word "should" and shove it down the garbage disposal. Whenever we use "should," we give away all our power.

Self-empowering questions that you can instead ask yourself are, "What do I choose to do now? What will give me the greatest sense of joy and fulfillment?" Answer these questions honestly, and then choose your action. Later, if the answers to these questions change, then "shift gears" and change what you're doing. You are not forever bound to any commitment. Do what feels right in the moment. When that feeling changes, do something else.

**The Cosmos states clearly that it is not hard of hearing!** When you invoke something, it heard you the first time. Any further repetition is simply a projection of lack of self-trust. Repetitive affirmations are often abused as a mental regurgitation of fear-based control. Affirmations and positive thinking can certainly help achieve clarity and identify patterns of negative expectations or rigid thinking. However, excessive dependence upon affirmations and positive thinking — especially in the absence of true emotional feeling and ownership — will lead to mental blockages and escape from the real emotional issues.

Be clear in what you desire. Let your desire fully permeate your emotional body. Allow the passion of your emotional body to fill up your physical body. Live your passion to the fullest by choosing actions which bring your dreams into manifestation. Then let life mirror to you whether this is for your true highest good. By living fully and completely in the moment, you will soon discover if a given path you have chosen is the one most appropriate to your current situation.

Just because we don't get what we want doesn't mean we can't have it. To open up to love, we must first open up to everything within us that is contrary to love. In reality, there is nothing contrary to love; but if we believe that love has an opposite, we create contrariness within us. When we open up to love, we must also open up to all the thoughts, fears, beliefs and expectations that block or deny true love before we can manifest our highest choice. So if something that we want doesn't come, or if it doesn't come in the way we want, or in the timing we want, this does not mean that we can't have it or that we are doing things wrong. Life simply mirrors that we have to resolve something within us that is contrary to love, something that we need to feel, own, and clear before we can move towards accepting what we truly want in our lives.

Vows come out of a sense of unworthiness and distrust. Commitment is not a vow. A vow is a mental projection based on doubt. Commitment is a deep feeling of self-being. We do not need vows to make commitments. If you are committed to self-healing and self-growth, ask yourself how to achieve this and then do it. Life will then mirror the inner blockages for you to meet and work with.

Again, ask yourself in any moment, "What do I feel? What does this feeling show me about myself? What do I choose to do with it?" Repeatedly asking and answering these questions helps you recognize the expectations, attitudes, beliefs and fears that must come up so you can own them without judging or fearing them. This process will naturally manifest your heart's desires.

## Vow of Chastity

The vow of chastity comes from the self-judgment of being inadequate and unworthy of love and also from the expectation of being rejected or abandoned by someone else. Most humans to a greater or lesser degree have subconscious imprinting from other life experiences that associate love with heartbreak and pain. We've all had lifetimes in which we were raped or in some other way sexually abused, as well as experiences of being the rapist and abuser. Also, many of us hold guilt for using our sexual power in past lives to lure other souls into our control. We used our sexual power to acquire greater wealth and power. Our pain and guilt from these experiences often led us to punish ourselves by taking vows of chastity.

The Universe does not require us to deny our sexual energy or to give up intimate relationships. In fact, we cannot fully experience ourselves unless we fully embrace our sexuality. You may choose chastity because that is what you truly desire. Then do so. But vows are imposed by self-limiting belief systems that mirror our fear to meet our own emotional denials.

There is tremendous guilt in vows made in relationships, particularly in marriages. In most religions a marriage is a holy vow, and to break that vow is a sin against God. The Cosmos does not recognize this God we believe we are sinning against. The best thing we can do is to commit ourselves as fully as possible to any relationship, then live and experience that relationship as totally and honestly as possible.

Not all relationships are meant to last forever. It is best to not place time limits on any relationship. Be in the relationship as fully and completely as possible in each moment. Allow yourself to feel and experience what it mirrors to you. Communicate as directly and honestly as possible. The relationship lasts for however long is best.

The end of a relationship is not a failure, and it is not the breaking of a sacred vow. It simply means you are ready to move on to another experience in order to receive other mirroring to get in touch with whatever emotions or experiences were not derived from the previous relationship. Or perhaps that relationship achieved such a completion that you are simply ready to move on to a totally different experience. Oftentimes the lesson in an abusive relationship is to love and honor and value ourselves enough to remove ourselves from the abuse and not remain out of some false sense of commitment.

The same goes for relationships between family members. People do not have to like each other or fulfill any obligations simply because they are blood relations. We co-create the family we are born into because each family member mirrors issues to the others. We can relate or not relate to each other according to how we feel in any moment. The point is to see ourselves in each family member; to own what is there for us to learn; to respect the other family members for who they are, and allow them to live their truth. If their truth is abusive to us, then the loving thing to do is to remove ourselves from the situation.

Blood may be thicker than water, but Spirit is thickest of all, and it requires no limiting vows or obligations. True commitment comes from a sense of recognizing and being ourselves fully in owning who we are. It is inconsequential whether a commitment to any person or thing lasts one minute, one year, a lifetime, or a million lifetimes. Commitment is not measured in quantity of time but rather by quality of being.

## Vow of Poverty

The vow of poverty is based on a belief in our own worthlessness. This belief in worthlessness is a punishment we chose to put upon ourselves due to past-life guilt for power abuse. We tried to convince ourselves that if we made ourselves less, then the power would be less, and therefore the consequences of the misuse of power would be less. Misuse of power is a vital learning tool to reflect back to us our own lack of self-love and self-trust. We lack trust in ourselves as unique spiritual beings, and misuse of power is an experience to show us that power is abused only because of lack of self-love. When we are ready to accept this truth, we can clear our attachment to *what* happens and focus on the *why* behind the action, for this is where our true growth and purpose exist.

No matter what abuse of power has been experienced on this planet, it is an expression of denied self-love. That is the purpose of those experiences. What happens or what doesn't happen is not the point. It is why we chose that experience, what we felt in the choosing and what we felt in the experience that is of significance. If we don't choose to take conscious responsibility to own our creative power, one form of escape is to focus on the *what*, judge it and get lost in emotional reactions based on the judgment.

Taking a vow of poverty is a way of ensuring struggle on the physical level to control power. The vow of poverty *screams* addiction to judging external events to avoid the real feelings that motivate and create them. When we are able to accept why any situation is happening (and the answer to that is always in our feelings), then we are able to move forward. The Universe does not require poverty for us to serve, heal or grow. Poverty stems from lack of self-worthiness and the blockage of energy flow that results from that self-judgment. To think that we are more spiritual or somehow closer to God by denying prosperity is a twisted tornado to keep our power limited and yet still feel spiritual. Our challenge is to be ourselves one hundred per cent and express that however we choose.

Money is just a symbol of energy flow, and energy flows in direct proportion to our attitude and acceptance of ourselves. It does not, however, automatically mean that the more we love ourselves, the more money we have, or the less money we have, the less we love ourselves. We could be living on very little money and not be living in poverty. By the same token, we could be multi-millionaires and live in absolute emotional and spiritual poverty. Poverty has nothing to do with amount of money but rather the abundance or lack of abundance of self-love and self-trust.

Money is not a cure-all, nor should it always be taken literally as a one-to-one reflection of our worthiness. It is simply that whether we have a lot of money or not, if we feel insecure that we don't have what we think we need or we don't have what it takes to accomplish our goals, this is a poverty of self-love. The presence or absence of money may not necessarily help or hinder the physical solutions. We look at the flow of money in our lives and ask what the mirror is and how the energy flows or doesn't flow within us. We can achieve greatness with little or no money, and we may achieve nothing with all the money in the Universe. The issue is to feel our sense of worthiness which is not dependent upon what we have, know or do.

Use emotional feeling to connect with the identification to money as self-value. If we value ourselves according to what we have or don't have, this is an external addiction that results in financial crisis. When we can accept that we do not have to earn love, or prove ourselves worthy of love, and our validation as a being is not dependent upon what we do or have, then we are on the path to embracing true self-worthiness.

A vow of poverty blocks us from this process. It results from externalizing God and therefore being cut off from our sense of self-love and self-worthiness. Humankind abused religion to externalize God in order to control power and avoid further abuse of power. This guilt-ridden illogic has only created more and more misuse of power and money.

When we truly love, honor and trust our own God-Selves, we don't need to do anything to prove ourselves and we don't need other people to believe in any particular ways. Then the vow of poverty is seen for what it is: a projection of self-worthlessness. When we are ready to accept that we do not need to give up anything to be our true selves and that we do not validate or measure ourselves by what we have, then we embody our true worthiness.

## Vow of Obedience

What is the point of doing what God tells us to do just because God tells us to do it? Do we truly envision God as a supreme puppet-master getting off on pulling strings? It has been stated beautifully before in Neale Donald Walsch's book *Conversations with God* that we were never given the "Ten Commandments" but rather the "Ten Commitments." Nothing is achieved if we do something because we are commanded. There is no external God doing anything *to* us. We are all God, even though we may not believe it, act like it or feel like it. Nevertheless, we are all God Totality and our unique individual selves simultaneously.

We are not talking here about the obedience a child should show a parent, but rather the vow of blind obedience adults choose to give to churches, military or any other individual or group. Certainly there are many appropriate situations for obedience in work situations, military defense, family, schools, etc. We refer only to extreme vows of obedience adults make that eventually lead to blind and destructive behaviors.

We are here to be ourselves one hundred per cent. Therefore, we are under no one's commands. The vow of obedience is a projection of not wanting to take responsibility for power because of past-life guilt about misuse of power. This begins to sound redundant, doesn't it? But there it is. So much of our beliefs, thoughts and reactions are based on this terror of power because we hold on to judgment of past misuse of power. Again, the perception of misuse of power was necessary to teach us that it resulted from lack of self-love. Obedience does not come out of love. Obedience comes from a mental projection of the need to escape self-ownership.

When we do anything for ourselves or others, it should come out of our deepest intuitive feelings. Do something because it feels right. Even when we commit to someone or something, commitment must contain flexibility of attunement to any given moment, and to the trusting and honoring of that attunement. Obedience blocks this kind of inner attunement. It turns us into robots. If we choose to give away our power so that someone else is responsible, then certainly we turn into robots. We shaped religion and society to run our lives so that we could give up as much responsibility and power as possible in exchange for being taken care of and being saved. When this didn't work, the very structures we had created instead became mirrors of excuse and blame.

Look at the heartlessness that religious groups have relentlessly acted out toward each other throughout history. Look at the wars that countries and ethnic groups have waged against each other. We see in this a pattern of robot consciousness. To serve in a church structure, an army or a political hierarchy requires someone to be the puppet master and everyone else to be the puppets. This is how life mirrors back to us the consequence of denying the responsibility of our power.

The vow of obedience is a fuel that feeds this destructive flame. If we are committed to our own truth and have an attuned sense of what is right for us in any given moment, then we are aligned with our truest spiritual selves for the highest good to manifest in our lives. Obedience strips away this opportunity. We are not bound by any vow of obedience to anyone or anything in this Universe. Our life challenge is to allow ourselves to feel and be however we choose in any given moment.

## Vow of Humility

It is now time to directly connect to our Higher Selves and listen to the truths from our own Inner Beings. It may not be immediately apparent why it is necessary to rescind a vow of humility because we have become so firmly entrenched into various religions that say it is good to be humble. This is dis-empowering and contributes greatly to a loss of self-esteem.

Our Creator wants us to be in our power at all times. By being humble, we diminish our sense of power and give in to outside authority figures. We are meant to be our own authority. We don't need to be limited by church doctrine which seeks to keep us under its control. Nor do we require self-diminishing humbleness in order to feel gratitude, respect, equality and love. Being humble is not the opposite of egotism. On the contrary, humility is often a direct expression of egotism, judging others as selfish or egotistical while believing ourselves to be superior in our imposed position of inferiority.

Humility is a word that has long had much judgment and misunderstanding projected into it. Let's clear this up now. The misuse of the vow of humility results in making us less than who we are. It denies our true God-being. When we project and externalize God, one result is seeing ourselves as separate and less. The Universe does not require us to be less. It does not wish for us to be separate from God. *All That Is by Its very nature is in an eternal state of expansion.* This expansion is hampered when we put ourselves down by believing or feeling ourselves to be less. There is no external God with a megalomaniacal ego needing to feel "superior" to Its "inferior" mortal souls. These beliefs are solely humanity's judgmental projections onto God.

If we re-define the word humility, we may tap into something very powerful. In this way, there is a concept of humility that is supportive and appropriate. This new definition of humility brings a feeling of recognizing the totality that exists within us, and at the same time realizing that the same totality exists equally in all beings and things. True humility involves honoring and loving that truth. It can also express itself as awe in the beauty and wonder of the Universe. Humility then means feeling respect and wonder, but not feeling superior or inferior to anything in manifestation.

The problem is, we try to use the same word for these two different concepts. It would be better to create a new word for this state of loving awareness and acceptance that does not require us to be less.

Meanwhile, our vows of humility can be cleared. We are closer to God the more we experience our totality of expression. To love ourselves and recognize ourselves as God does not mean that we see ourselves as superior to anyone. Self-love is not egotistical. People who are egotistical do not love themselves. A superior attitude is a cover up used to suppress a deeply denied feeling of inferiority. So do not confuse egotism with self-love or knowing that you are God.

Part of the vow of humility is this belief that the power is "not of me, but comes through me." To that we say, "Horse manure!" Any power, healing energy, inspiration or intuition that we experience not only comes through us but *is us*! So let's stop separating ourselves from our power, skills and abilities. The false humility that the power is not us is a rejection of self-truth and self-love. This concept can be released along with the vow of humility itself.

We will now make a list of other vows that some souls may have made in various lifetimes. Check if any of these apply to you. If so, then rescind them if you are complete with the experiences you have had while maintaining these vows.[2]

## Other Vows

- Allegiance to any club, secret society or organization
- Allegiance to any race or country
- Promising to *never* leave a person, to *always* "be there" for a person
- All marriages or relationship vows to significant others
- Vows made to children, brothers, sisters, friends
- Vows made to a profession ("I'll be a healer for all time and eternity")
- All legal contracts
- Vows to correct all justice causes in regards to a particular race, nationality or geographical region
- Vows to not do one thing until we have completed something else ("I won't have a personal relationship until I have righted this wrong in regards to my father")
- Vows to avenge a perceived wrong
- Always being close to those we love and being very far away from those we identify as the enemy

[2] Love, respect and commitment do not require formal vows and need to come from the heart rather than from guilt-ridden and judgmentally pressuring formal vows.

## Vows We Made to Ourselves

In many lifetimes, we have had experiences with men or women which were painful. We may have made a vow to *never* have another relationship with the opposite sex; to *only* have a relationship with one particular sex; to avoid sexual relationships; to only incarnate as a woman, or only as a man. We may wonder why we don't have a "significant other." If you had a painful relationship in one or more lifetimes and vowed to yourself to never get involved ever again in a relationship, it is no wonder why you are unable to attract someone special to you.

You may have had lifetimes in which you were a particular race and there were unfavorable situations involved in that race, or in that part of the world, or both. You may have made vows to *never* or *always* be a particular race, or to live or not live in a particular part of the world. Perhaps due to your work, you now find yourself a Chinese woman living in America, having a challenging time creating a wonderful, intimate relationship. Perhaps you vowed to come into this lifetime as a Chinese woman, to be a path cutter for women's rights. So, you chose to come to America to interact with other women doing similar things. Maybe this is working out well for you in the area of women's rights and freedoms. Yet, the intimate relationship eludes you. Maybe you made a vow to not have a relationship until you had achieved something in your career. Discovering inherent vows in life situations such as these can assist in your choice to break free of those vows in order to be more in the present moment and create the life situations you truly desire.

## Karma & Other Feelings of Obligation

Many of us feel obligations to people we have spent time with in other life experiences. Perhaps a friend saved our life or did us a big favor in the past. Perhaps someone made a big sacrifice at his or her expense and we feel an obligation to repay that debt. Perhaps we took advantage of someone in another lifetime, and we now find ourselves endlessly giving to this person without knowing why.

Karma has many misconceptions associated with it. Some traditions teach that we must pay back *in equal and full measure* for every action we ever did. If we killed someone, we must be killed. If we stole, we must pay back every penny of that, plus interest. If we raped, abused or harmed others, then we must endure harm to our physical bodies until that debt is paid in full.

Karma is an energy that is here to teach us. Its purpose is not to punish us for past actions but to facilitate learning through ownership and responsibility of action. Maybe we did kill 300 people in some past lifetimes, but that doesn't mean we have to in return be killed 300 times. It just means that we need to learn not to kill ever again. Maybe it only took us 20 times of being killed to learn this lesson. So be it. Self-forgiveness for what we did is a key to accepting self-responsibility, learning a lesson and moving on.

There are no victims. If we did kill someone, perhaps they felt they needed that experience to balance something in them for their soul's growth. God always matches up those who choose to inflict damage with those who feel they need damage inflicted upon them until both recognize they are two sides of the same coin called "self-denial," mirroring each other in order to learn the same lesson.

There is a subtle level of karma that is often overlooked. As we learn, grow and evolve, we are then responsible for our choices on a much higher level. In the case of killing, we soon realize that it is also unloving to kill people's ideas, dreams and passions. This is far more "deadly" to the spirit than killing someone's physical body.

## Curses & Hexes

We choose to invoke a curse or hex as a way of projecting our own disgust, pain, fear or hurt onto others. Thus, giving, as well as receiving, curses and hexes are actually distorted cries for self-love.

The atmosphere of Mother Earth, like the auras of human bodies, is clogged with unresolved curses and hexes. This is a manifestation of humanity's need to take full ownership and responsibility for its self-creative experiences. With the religious vows we saw how we give away our energies through promises that ultimately strip us of power, love and self-worth. With curses and hexes, we project onto another in an act of hurtful vengeance that denies our self-responsibility and which will, in the end, only cause us the equal self-pain and struggling that we invoked upon the other.

When we create or request a hex to wreak revenge, get money or make someone fall in love with us, we are acting out our feelings of low self-worth. Creating a love potion, for example, to force someone to fall in love with us reflects back to past lifetime experiences of lovelessness, loneliness, and rejection by others. The ramifications of such an act is not a punishment from the Universe, because the Universe neither judges nor punishes. It is simply the reflected consequence of trying to force another into an action, situation or feeling not of their conscious choosing.

A hex cannot influence another unless that individual chooses to believe in the power of the hex. When we are in a state of absolute ownership of our own emotions and creative processes, we do not absorb another's hex into our energy fields or experiences. Those who believe in the reality of a hex can become the "victimized" recipients to show them that believing in the power of the hex is, in reality, a self-imposed hex. People receive hexes and curses because they are consciously or unconsciously judging and punishing themselves for past perceived misuses of power. Thus they draw the curses and hexes to them so they can cease judging and punishing themselves and instead accept what these experiences reveal about their own self-perceptions.

Curses that are placed on whole families, cultures, nations and races have only the degree of power that the collective consciousness of that group chooses to accept. Oftentimes, we incarnate into one group or another that has had a curse imposed upon it because this mirrors to us the false beliefs that we choose to give power to.

If you feel you have placed curses or hexes on individuals or groups in other life experiences, it is important to get in touch with what emotions surround that choice, and what feelings or experiences would drive you to invoke a curse or a hex upon another. Do so with a willingness to not place further guilt, criticism, judgment or punishment upon yourself. Acknowledge and accept whatever emotional memories, fears or denials are triggered by this this process. If you feel you have placed curses or hexes in any past life, you can now set the energies free which have been held in the curse or hex. This will involve feeling a deep forgiveness for yourself while embracing whatever emotions surface as part of the releasing of the curse or hex. Again, do not impose any further guilt or self-judgment. Gratefully accept what the experience illustrates about your own fears and self-denials and embrace whatever emotions come to the surface. In doing so, you can heal the emotional pain that created the initial curse or hex and neutralize any manifestation of the curse or hex in this present moment.

If you feel you had a curse or hex placed upon you by others, go within to discover why you chose to believe in the reality of the curse or hex. Why do you feel you deserve a curse or hex? How does this make you feel? What does this feeling tell you about your perception or definition of yourself? Finally, what do you choose to do with this perception or definition?

Allowing this inner journey of discovery, you can choose to no longer believe in or give power to curses or hexes. In owning and honoring the emotions surrounding these judgments, you are ready to clear away all beliefs in or need for curses or hexes. Be thankful for the learning experience and let go of the need to be a victim of a curse or hex. This will erase the curses or hexes you hold in the cellular memories of your physical body.

Some people choose to have a more tangible ritualistic experience to feel the reality of releasing curses and hexes, whether they were the giver or the recipient. So long as we accept that the ritual itself is not really the power but rather a symbolic reflection of the power within us, then the ritual can be a powerful experience to help us achieve emotional healing and cleansing.

**Here is a suggested ritual:** Light three candles: pink (forgiveness), white (integration of experiences and lessons) and violet (purification and release). Burn Sage and circulate the burning Sage over your head, on all sides of yourself and in every corner of every room of your home. Also burn Sandalwood and Frankincense along with the three candles. You may also want to diffuse the essential oils of Sage, Sandalwood, Cedarwood or Spruce.

Sit or lay down in front of the candles and incense with a rose quartz in your left hand and an amethyst in your right hand. The rose quartz represents forgiveness and the violet amethyst represents purification and clearing. If you feel that the curse or hex is intensely strong, use dark green jade over you heart chakra to open you to the pure love essence of your being. It can be worn as a necklace or as a solitary stone.

Visualize the curse or hex (whether you are the giver or recipient) as a color and/or shape in your auric field. For some people this may be one vast black hole, and for others it may be many small holes or rents in their aura. Some people visualize faces, animals or beings in their aura as representations of these energies. Then allow yourself to feel fully whatever emotions come to you when you focus on the symbolic manifestations of this energy. Accept and honor these emotions as the true initial feelings that caused you to believe in the curse or hex. Then invoke from your heart true self-forgiveness and a conscious choice to no longer believe or accept these energies.

For some people carrying out this ritualistic invocation only once may achieve a full completion. For others it may be necessary to repeat the ritual several times until they see and feel a complete absence of the dark holes, rents or other symbolic manifestations in their auras. Eventually you will feel a sense of completion, an absence of these energies and a sense of loving acceptance and wholeness. This will be your inner confirmation that you are complete with this ritualistic experience.

This ritual can be done in silence or accompanied by music. If you choose to use music, we recommend Celtic harp music or classical concertos of stringed instruments. Many of the violin concertos were specifically channeled through the classical composers for emotional healing and spiritual integration. Particularly powerful as musical accompaniment in these ritualistic purifications are: the violin concertos of Bruch, Beethoven, Tchaikovsky, Mendelssohn and Dvorak; the Sixth Symphony (*Pathetique*) by Tchaikovsky; the soundtrack from the film *Chariots of Fire* by Vangelis; the Celtic harp music of Alan Stivell entitled *Renaissance of the Celtic Harp*; and any music by Enya or Loreena McKennitt.

It is also greatly beneficial for many people after experiencing a purification to soak for 15-20 minutes in a tub of hot water with essential oils to help the body clear out the emotional issues that have surfaced. After soaking in the tub, lay down in bed. Rather than drying yourself off, simply wrap yourself in a towel or robe and rest for at least half an hour to allow the body to process the emotional and energetic clearings. Here, too, the above-mentioned music can be used as part of this integrating process.

The essential oils[3] that best assist you in processing this deep emotional clearing of curses and hexes are: Rose, Lavender, Sage, Sandalwood, Cedarwood, Cypress, Birch and Cinnamon, as well as these essential oil blends: Purification, Release, Forgiveness, Peace & Calming, Joy and 3 Wise Men.

The existence of curses and hexes illustrate the importance of taking full responsibility and ownership for all of our life experiences. No one makes us feel or do anything. We are not

[3] Contact Dr. Foley for assistance in using Essential Oils.

victims of a victimizing world. No one can have any power over us except what we choose to give them.

Curses and hexes also teach us not to blame anyone for our experiences and to totally own our power. They exist as an opportunity to forgive all self-creative choices and to honor the true lessons they illustrate about denial of self-love. Everything we perceive as negative actions against us are really just projections of self-hatred and self-fear. When we stop blaming and accusing one another for mirroring our self-denied issues, then the unresolved curse and hex energies can be cleansed.

## Psychic Cording

Any time we feel a strong connection with anyone or anything, this forms an energetic bonding known as psychic cording. It is an energy based on pure perception and has whatever power we give it. Psychic cording can have a positive or negative quality and is created by an intense feeling of unity with another being, place, idea or thing.

Many of us have idealistically romantic perceptions of soul mates, twin souls or twin flames. Certainly there is a strong energy linking those who share many lifetime experiences together or who share particularly intense life experiences, (which is neither good nor bad). But often the resulting psychic cording will cause a repetition of the experience. This will then bring forth strong energies of memory, emo tional reaction and desire that can have many levels of effects upon us.

The term "soul mate" refers to incarnate spiritual entities who share several emotionally charged experiences in various lifetimes. Soul mates therefore repeatedly magnetize to each other and will often consciously or subconsciously recognize the highly charged vibrations between their auric energies.

It is not true that all soul mates, twin souls or twin flames automatically love one another passionately, unconditionally and infinitely. Soul mates are not automatically friendly to each other. Intensely "negative" experiences can draw spiritual beings together as soul mates. The romantic New Age notion that being soul mates implies an automatically loving relationship denies the reality of "negative" memories that are often being acted out. Sometimes it is for the highest good that soul mates *not* get along lovingly. It is important to recognize the healing potential of "negative" experiences rather than to hold on to the belief that soul mates must be automatically loving or blissful with each other.

"Twin souls" or "twin flames" are interchangeably used to refer to two individuals who are simultaneously incarnated facets of the same Higher Self energy. Soul mates, twin souls and twin flames are not always automatically partnered as male and female. Many twin souls or twin flames are paired as male/male or female/female, as well as being male/female. When we have an immediate "recognition" of someone (whether positive or negative), an energetic cording is being awakened that connects the present incarnate experience to unresolved lessons and emotional processes from other lifetimes. It is important to not get carried away by or addicted to the phenomenon of experiencing this magnetic cording, but rather to simply recognize the feeling as a confirmation of a soul we have magnetized to us in the moment for something we choose to experience and complete. It is best to not project any assumption of positive or negative results, no matter how this magnetic cording feels to us, so as not to manipulate, distort or prevent the fuller spectrum of experience that can be shared in this present lifetime. Furthermore, it is important to not hold on to the sensation of this cording as any kind of validation of experience, but to release that feeling when and if the shared experience is completed and it is time to move on to other relationships and experiences.

Feeling drawn to certain buildings or geographical locations on the planet is another manifestation of psychic cording. This is often a confirmation that we have been in this building or place in another lifetime. It can be a positive exercise in recognizing self-communication from a higher level of consciousness. Beyond that, it is important to not attach any more idealistic meaning or addiction to this kind of experience. Once the recognition is made, we embrace it, appreciate it and move on.

We also experience a form of psychic cording by holding on to particular ideas, beliefs, perceptions or expectations from one life experience to another. It is important to challenge ourselves in a completely nonjudgmental way about why we choose to believe, think, perceive or expect what we do. This way, we can be clear about what our truth is, what we choose our truth to be, and why we make the choices we do.

Guilt, judgment, blame, negative expectation, victimization and the unwillingness to forgive ourselves or others all maintain a self-destructive psychic cording with other individuals and belief systems. When we recognize that all life experience is self-created to enable us to learn and grow, we can then accept that we magnetize to us certain individuals and experiences in order to mirror our issues and trigger our emotions. This self-forgiveness and self-grace then results in our severing unproductive psychic cordings.

Pay special attention to those you choose as your parents. For example, we choose parents who most directly mirror our perceptions of our own masculine and feminine energies. We also choose parents who mirror our ideas of God the Father and God the Mother. The psychic bonding with our parents is therefore of particular importance in our self-discovery and inner-ownership. Once we see and accept what our parents mirror to us about our own attitudes and feelings regarding our masculine and feminine energies as well as our ideas of the Godhead, we can then forgive any "negative" experiences with our parents and move into a state of self-ownership that allows us to relate to them as unique individuals without the distorted psychic cordings of blame, guilt and victimization.

If we experience the death or separation from one or both parents before reaching adulthood, this is often a symbolic indication that our masculine or feminine energies are being cut off in our conscious development. The death or disappearance of a father often indicates a severe lack of connection with our masculine energies. By the same token, the death or disappearance of a mother would indicate a severe denial of feminine energies. The younger we are at the time of death or disappearance of a parent, the more intense the issue and most probably the more severe the history of the pattern.

Having both parents separated from us indicates a kind of limbo consciousness where we may be so severely out of touch with both masculine and feminine energies that our life experience tends to be one of aimless, unconscious reactions to life rather than a conscious capacity for true creative experience. Often we choose to experience a life as an orphan if we have been so caught up in identifying ourselves with our family history that we have no sense of our true spiritual selves, or else we have acted out a pattern of aimless victimization in many lifetimes and now choose to have an experience that will help us find an anchor of self-identity that is not dependent on the direct history and mirroring of the family into which we were born.

The psychic cord between child and parents can still remain strong even when a parent or both parents are absent due to death or abandonment. There can still be strong emotional connections at the dream-state level or in the body's cellular memory. It is not unusual for the dead or missing parent to become a spirit guide maintaining the psychic cord while the child experiences (parental) mirroring through other individuals.

Adoptive, foster or step-parents also act as mirrors for the masculine and feminine issues of the child and have their own psychic cording distinct from the original parents. Here again, we choose these situations to discover a deeper self-identity.

Whoever acts in our lives as a parental figure also mirrors things of the masculine and feminine issues we need to recognize and own. As we have indicated, even the physical absence of a parent can still energetically charge a psychic cording if that absence will stimulate the issues more powerfully than if the original parent were present. Where there are both original parents and step-parents in the picture, this often indicates a further fragmentation in the history of a child's relationship to its masculine and feminine issues (depending on which parent or parents are involved) that require the added mirrors to illustrate the fragmentation and the opportunity to recognize and heal the emotional issues being acted out between us and the adults.

In the same way, mirroring works with our siblings, children, lovers, friends, work associates and even our "enemies." Whatever we love the most in another is what we most love within ourselves. Whatever we dislike or hate the most in another is what we judge as most disgusting within ourselves. This creates psychic cording that ties us to the other until our self-revelations and emotional ownerships are totally experienced and embodied. Only then can the psychic bonds be cut so that we can relate to each other more purely as unique individuals.

The physical absence of children, siblings, lovers, and friends (whether by death, abandonment or any other reason) mirrors our denial of whatever emotional qualities these individuals represent to us. We can ask ourselves, "What quality do I think of and feel when I focus on this child, sibling, lover, etc.?" The answer reveals the qualities they mirror to us, and we can then start the process of owning and feeling those issues.

## Those Who Live Alone

As useful as it is to see what our spouse or children mirror to us, it is also important to recognize what is going on in those who don't have a lot of people in their lives. People often say, "I'd rather have no relationship than have dysfunctional ones." Yes, there is wisdom in this statement. We are free to live alone and not have husbands, wives and children.

There is nothing wrong with choosing to have a quiet life without a partner or a family. Sometimes a person gets married, raises children and then chooses to live alone. This is neither better or worse than choosing to have a partner. *It all depends upon the intention of each person.* Some people use this solitary experience to process deep emotional imprints and they simply choose the peace and solitude of this way of life.

If one has just had a painful breakup, it can be healthy to live alone for a period of time for self-reflection. Those who continually put themselves in relationships without healing from the last one can run away within relationships. This way they can conveniently focus on the other person rather than to look inside. Some people live alone as a way of hiding out, so they don't have to look in the mirror and see the reflections other people would have given them. This often leads to greater challenges with co-workers and neighbors instead, as they try to avoid painful reflections by not having any more intimate relationships.

It is easier to avoid conflicts if we live alone. However, most of us came to this planet and this third dimension to work through our challenges, not run away from them. While it is sometimes more painful, it can also be much more rewarding to learn together with others. We grow much more quickly while engaged in each others energies.

There are no rules here, as each situation is different. What is important is to feel into your motivations, your intentions and to pay attention to any patterns which may exist. Closely monitor your present relationships, or lack thereof, to discover what is true for you.

## Abortions & Miscarriages

To those who believe abortion is murder, we certainly understand why they choose to view it that way. However, we suggest that it is impossible to kill Spirit. Any form of death, abortion or otherwise, is just a transition from one state of consciousness to the next.

Many people *claim* to reject abortion because it is murder. Some truly feel this way, but many only mouth the words. Intense denial is being played out around abortion – the denial that many human souls are actually threatened by a woman having power and authority over her own life and body.

The Universe is neither pro nor con abortion. Every incarnate spirit has the responsibility for self-authority and choice, even if they choose to not realize it. To be a fundamentalist of any religious or political belief is to surrender our self-authority and choice to a belief system. Much of the controversy around abortion is actually about this and not about the life or death of the fetus. There is no such thing as death – only the perceived experience of it. To not accept this can feed the fear of death and therefore the need to relinquish choice and authority to someone else.

Karmically, a woman chooses abortion or miscarriage for many reasons: (1) She has had past-life experience of dying in childbirth; (2) She remembers her children repeatedly dying at very early ages; (3) She remembers struggling and suffering while attempting to raise her families; (4) She feels incapable of raising the child; (5) She lacks the maturity or desire to bear the responsibility of motherhood; or (6) there is severe disharmony between her masculine and feminine energies.

Abortion and miscarriages often indicate a woman's lack of awareness, appreciation or faith in her own masculine energy. To reject bringing a baby to full development and birth can teach a woman to recognize and honor her own masculine qualities of courage, strength and self-authority in acting on her conscious choices.

Much of this blockage of a woman's masculine energy derives from lifetimes of domination, control and abuse by imbalanced men. Rape, incest, physical and emotional abuse, and severely painful childbirths can create an emotionally charged energy field that settles in the womb and sexual organs. Built up over many lifetimes, this can cause the experiences of abortions and miscarriages. Regression Therapy, Rebirthing, Akashic Readings, Body Massage and Dream Therapy can assist in exploring past-life experiences and the suppressed emotional memories that can feed abortion choices.

Sometimes incarnate spirits have experienced a long succession of lifetimes as women brainwashed into believing their *only* value and purpose is to bear children (often as many as possible) and to raise families. With this severe denial of self-value, it can be very valuable for these souls to experience saying "no" to pregnancy, marriage and family responsibilities in order to recapture a truer sense of self that does not depend on what society expects of them.

The impact of abortions and miscarriages goes beyond the woman to the father, the other children, the grandparents, all relatives and all members of society. Experiencing death through abortion or miscarriage triggers emotions of loss and grief in the present moment as well as from other lifetimes. The people involved are then faced with the choice of embracing and healing these emotions, or to deny and bury them until next time.

Like ripples in the water caused from a falling stone, an abortion or miscarriage can help many people get in touch with their fear-based beliefs about life, death, purpose and self-value. We *all* have "aborted" or "miscarried" dreams, projects, desires and relationships due to laziness, fear, restrictive beliefs, judgmental expectations or the most common excuse of all, "What will the neighbors think?" All souls continually abort and miscarry self-love, trust, passion and the willingness to dare. We use our fears of other people's reactions as an excuse to deny what we most desire.

Abortions and miscarriages reveal a disharmony between the masculine and feminine energies within the woman. They also mirror to everyone around her their own lack of commitment to their innermost truths, dreams and desires.

To be a fundamentalist (or judgmentalist!) of any religious or political belief system is the ultimate self-abortion. We cannot be true to our emotions, intuition, dreams, desires and innermost God-Self if an external God or savior is the sole source of truth and authority. This is one reason why fundamentalists so aggressively oppose abortion or anything outside their rigid belief structure. A woman having total choice and authority over her own life and body threatens people who place all power and authority in a dogma and God outside of themselves. A woman in full power and control of her life violates the deepest self-denial of fundamentalism, and that is the *true* abortion.

Abortions and miscarriages also provide useful lessons for the potential incarnate spirit who does not achieve the physical birth at that time. Often, the incarnating soul experienced extreme trauma in a previous life, such as sudden or violent deaths, or long periods of abuse or torture. Sometimes these souls choose to prepare for a full incarnation by living for a short time within the mother's womb. This short life experience is akin to aversion therapy to overcome fear of spiders, for instance. In this type of therapy, a person has small exposures to what frightens them until they get used to it.

Sometimes a soul chooses a mother who is not going to have a full-term pregnancy. The soul may stay in the mother's womb for several months and decide that is enough, or it may change its mind about incarnating at this time.

Many souls who have died in concentration camps, wars, earthquakes, domestic violence or after severe illness, or those who caused death, violence or suffering to others, often fear rebirth and the negative expectation of "more of the same." This trauma can also feed into the experience of an abortion or miscarriage, requiring the soul to undergo deep self-evaluation, counseling and healing at other levels of reality before re-attempting their next physical incarnation.

Sometimes spirits volunteer to exist in the aura of a pregnant woman to facilitate the experience of an impending abortion or miscarriage. This is an opportunity for emotional healing and ownership for all those concerned. The volunteering spirit knows it will not physically incarnate at that time; but by helping others to feel and experience something that can help them grow, the non-incarnated spirit also derives understanding to help prepare it for its next eventual incarnation.

Another dimension of the drama of abortion concerns a particular soul's choice to incarnate in the first place through a particular physical entity — in other words, a child's choice of mother. All of us, before we incarnate, choose the setting into which we incarnate, sometimes through guilt and a wish to punish ourselves rather than as a choice of mature spiritual wisdom. We choose the culture and country in which to incarnate. We choose our family and relatives. And perhaps most important of all, we choose our mother and father.

A soul that fully respects the choice and will of other soul entities would normally not try to incarnate through a woman who does not want to become pregnant or have any children. So merely the fact that a woman gets pregnant against her own desire often indicates that a soul is trying to come onto the Earth plane who has the capacity to override the will of other souls. However, every case is unique and we do not mean to make this an absolute statement.

Sometimes mother and child may have agreed on such a learning experience beforehand on another level of reality, and the mother has just forgotten the agreement. Or, the child might have chosen the experience in order to work on healing issues about feeling unloved, unwanted or unworthy. The mother could have unconsciously chosen the experience in order to face responsibilities and challenges she wouldn't have had the courage to choose consciously.

The only thing that is certain is that on some level both mother and child (as well as the father) choose the experience, either out of guilt or emotional denials, or to have a precious learning experience together. However, in order to fully understand the complex issue of abortion and pro-choice vs. pro-life, it is important to be aware that some souls who incarnate through an unwanted pregnancy may have no scruples about overrunning the will of other people.

The conscious choice of a woman to have an abortion may also increase her strength in the area of her masculine, discerning, self-loving energies. Sometimes to choose abortion is also to choose not to let comparatively heartless and inconsiderate souls enter the Earth plane. However, every case is unique and please do not base your decision to have an abortion on any one thing we say in this book. Instead use loving self-reflective discernment to make the important decision of bringing a particular soul to Earth. Use your emotional body to feel the essence of the unborn child's soul. Do you feel love for the child? Does the child have any love and respect for you as its parent?

All souls are love. The souls who try to incarnate through a woman against her will are not less so, but they are in more denial of their true loving nature and therefore more prone to be inconsiderate and cause hurt and pain to others. We who are already on the Earth plane have the sovereign right to choose who to allow to incarnate and join us on this plane of existence, just as countries have the right to accept or refuse individuals who seek to immigrate.

Souls who go through with the experience of incarnating through a woman against her will are often the same people who end up being aggressively anti-abortion. The reason for this is very simple. These people do not love themselves and do not feel that anybody else could possibly love them. They subconsciously feel that in order to get anything in life, they have to take it by force without consideration of other people. This is not something they learned through a tough upbringing. It was imprinted in their souls before they were born. Often times, however, a tough upbringing will reinforce their already existing subconscious imprints, in accordance with the law that we attract experiences that mirror what's already inside of us.

So these incarnate souls entered the Earth plane by acquiring a physical body by force through an unwilling mother. As adults they do not consciously remember this choice, but the memory of it is alive in their subconscious minds. The power of women to choose abortions still feels literally life threatening to them. Basically these souls loathe themselves so deeply that they don't feel they deserve to live, unless the option exists for them to acquire a physical body by force of will.

Abortions and miscarriages are far more than what they appear to be. They are not the end of a life, but rather potentially powerful healing and learning experiences for all exposed to the experience, both those physically incarnated and those who remain in the etheric.

## Artificial Insemination & Test Tube Pregnancies

At the moment of conception, the embryo that is created receives a quantity and quality of life force through the orgasm of the father. The quantity and quality of the space that is opened to give the soul a place in the physical realm is determined by the orgasm of the mother. And the love that the mother and father feel for each other at the moment of conception fills the forming fetus with a quantity and quality of love-vibration. This is a very different picture than the one the scientists give us, where it's only a matter of an egg merging with a sperm.

Many people alive today were conceived without their mother even having an orgasm. That means there wasn't really any spiritual or emotional space opened for them to come into this world. So these souls often don't feel they have a place in this world. They don't feel they belong. They may become outcasts, homeless or bullies, caught in a web of external and/or internal aggression.

Of course, a man has to have an orgasm in order to ejaculate, so we're all born with some life-force from the orgasm our father had when he produced the sperm which provided 50% of our DNA. Again, the quantity and quality of the life force we were born with is determined by the intensity and nature of that orgasm.

However, when it comes to artificial insemination and test tube fertilization, there is usually no love whatsoever present between the mother and the genetic father at the moment of conception. So the embryo created this way receives no boost of love-vibration at its conception. A child symbolically and spiritually represents the heart between the mother and the father at the moment of conception. A child conceived without love between the mother and the genetic father will be a "heart" without any love present in it.

This is not a judgment, and as in the discussion before about abortions, we do not mean to condemn the children who were born in this manner. They may be souls who have never experienced the love-vibration within themselves and who have come to Earth to work on themselves and heal that emptiness within. They might have come here to help heal heartlessness on Earth. They could be of very loving intent, even if lacking in love.[4] Then again, they might not have loving intent in mind at all when they choose to incarnate here.

The same thing applies to the parents of the children we judge to be "loveless brats." Please do not use what we tell you in this book as a justification for your judgments of others or as a reason to beat others over the head. Each case is unique and has to be felt as such. We only tell you the information above to help you make "an informed decision," in case you're thinking of having a baby in either of these ways.

[4] Loving intent is a mental mindset different from love, which is a feeling.

## Disembodied Entities

It is important at this point to differentiate the terms "spirit" and "soul." When we use the term "spirit," we refer to the pure Life Force that is the truth of who you really are. "Soul" refers to an incarnate experience of any spiritual being. If you see yourself as a pearled necklace, each pearl represents an incarnate life experience that would be called a "soul." The string that connects all the pearls to make the unified necklace is the true pure living essence that we call "spirit." Thus, you are a Spiritual Being with many incarnate soul lifetimes.

Many times when a soul dies, the transition back to the original Spirit Source is disrupted by a trauma, fear or limiting belief system of denial. What is referred to as a "ghost" or "disembodied astral entity" is often a soul memory that is still tied to the Earth plane because of an intense emotional trauma or death that disrupted its complete re-integration back into its original Spirit Source. This phenomenon can manifest in varied levels of conscious awareness. Sometimes it is just a lingering emotional/energetic memory that repeats itself like a flashing light for a period of time until the intensity vibrates itself back to its Source. Other times there is a deeper state of consciousness attached to the energy resulting in a ghost who can interact with our physical reality, or as a disembodied astral entity trapped in a kind of no-man's land between the physical and etheric dimensions.

Some of these trapped entities are in severe fear and intend no harm to incarnate beings. They are simply lost in their own trauma, seeking guidance and light to free them of their transitional state so they can shift back to their Source. Other entities who are more present in their consciousness in this state of disembodiment and who have been extremely caught up in their fears, denials and physical addictions, often seek escape from their predicament by attempting to attach to the auric energies of incarnate souls.

A disembodied entity can only attach itself to the aura of a soul that is acting out deep levels of fear, guilt, self-condemnation, physical addictions or emotional denials. This is a profound learning tool to teach souls to take conscious responsibility for their lives and not choose to escape their life process through maintaining their denials. The more consciously we take ownership of our creative lives and of all our emotions, beliefs and choices, the more difficult it is for any disincarnate entity to attach to our auras and feed off our energies. If you think going to a healer or therapist to clear your auric field acting out some ritualistic procedure or taking any kind of medicines or treatments will sufficiently rid your aura of these entities, you still have much to learn. These entities know how to temporarily "step out" of our auras so that we appear to be cleared, and then "step back in" to our auras and resume feeding off our energies.

The only true healing of corded entities to our auras is a truthful commitment to our emotional ownership, which involves releasing the need to blame anyone for our creative choices or for choosing to see ourselves as victims of this world. When we can feel all our emotions as ours and honor them for what they show us about ourselves, this journey can lead us to the highest level of healing and expansion and also clear out any attached disincarnate entities.

We also state firmly at this point that there is no such thing as satanic possession. What we call Satan, the devil, demons, evil or dark forces are projections of our own self-hatred and self-denial. We are responsible for the self-destructive psychic cording we have created by choosing to invent religious beliefs that support the fiction that God is an exclusively external entity, and that there is a devil or dark forces that are also exclusively external to us. What we choose to believe, we create. Then we become addicted to acting out our belief systems by thinking life is validating our beliefs when, in actuality, life merely mirrors what we choose to believe.

Until we cease our pattern of externalizing our inner light and darkness as external beams, we are bound to live and re-live this experience like a snake swallowing its own tail. Eventually we need to spit that tail out and break the cycle through our willingness to accept and feel the reality that everything is us.

The more we intensify our fears, denials and beliefs into external entities, the more painful, demonic and dark they appear. This is not because that is the way they really are, but because that is the way we create them to appear so we have an excuse to run away and blame something outside of us for what is happening. What appears to us as evil or dark comes after us not because it wants to destroy us (although we manufacture it to look that way so we have an excuse to run and have something outside of us save us). This energy comes to us seeking our ownership and acceptance so that we may learn the real lesson it represents and thereby be healed. Then this psychic cording can be cleared away. This universal principle is beautifully illustrated in Ursula K. LeGuin's *Earthsea Trilogy*.

## Soul Fragments

Every time we deny and suppress an emotional experience, we energetically project out a fragment of our soul essence. This energy then merges with individuals around us who end up acting out our denied lesson or experience. The denied essence can also manifest itself as disease in our bodies. When we repeatedly deny and suppress emotional experiences life after life, these denials can build to such an intensity that they coalesce to become separately incarnated human individuals.

These incarnated soul fragments often live out lives of extreme suffering, such as dying of starvation or disease, or they manifest as humans of pure aggression and rage. Much of the suffering and violence on this planet is being acted out by those who are no more than incarnated manifestations of our denied guilt, fear, pain, grief or rage. These fragment-beings are often not open to understand or accept any other experience except what they are acting out. Humanity may complain about being victimized and bothered by the starving, by the relentless victims, and by the psychotically insane terrorists who continue to act out the same things over and over. What many do not understand is that these fragments will continue to act out our denials until we are willing to re-integrate as our own these denied and fragmented out emotions that we are afraid to feel, own or learn from within ourselves.

It is not enough to only send money, food, clothes and other forms of physical support to trouble spots on Earth. We must also understand that they mirror our projected denials that we refuse to recognize and own. Starvation in the world is a projected reflection of the spiritual and emotional starvation most souls experience but deny in themselves by escaping into addictions or rigid religious beliefs. Genocide and terrorism are manifestations of the guilt, judgment and denied self-rage humans do not own in themselves. We will continue to feel and act like victims until we show not only loving compassion for these fragment-souls but also a willingness to open our arms and hearts to accept these souls as reflections of ourselves.

Many people wonder if the world population has increased so vastly because there are so many newly created souls or so many other beings arriving from other worlds. The primary answer is that many, many people on Earth are fragments of denied emotional essence from other incarnated souls. Only when we accept that everything on Earth is a reflection of ourselves, our issues, our needs and our responsibilities will these fragments be absorbed back into their original Spirit Essence.

No one is an island. No one is a victim of a victimizing world. No one is going to be saved by an external God, an external savior, or by extra-terrestrials. We have the full responsibility to save ourselves by focusing on our emotions and by recognizing that all life is chosen and created by our innermost selves. We must also accept responsibility for recognizing and retrieving into our hearts the fragmentation of our own denials that have built up over so many lifetimes and have resulted in so many soul fragments running amok on the planet. We must eventually take full responsibility for our self-created world and stop looking for external saviors or external stimuli to escape the inner truth that is reflected back to us daily. We must strip away this distorted mask and see the truth that all of "them" are us.

# Chapter 3
# Emotional Ownership

The single most important reason for physical existence is to experience emotional ownership. This is our true ultimate mission on Earth. Most people think they are bound to Earth by an exclusively external mission of teaching or serving others. Certainly this is an aspect of it; but in actuality we are our own ultimate missions. We are in physical bodies to develop our emotional bodies and integrate them both fully into our spiritual being.

Emotional ownership means allowing ourselves to feel one hundred per cent any and all emotions and feelings, and to accept them one hundred per cent as our own creation. Many New Agers are trapped in the belief that they grow spiritually through mental learning and then doing external missions. However, our main spiritual growth does *not* come through knowing, understanding, learning or doing. Spiritual expansion primarily comes from feeling and being who we are to the absolute honest depth and being of our Selves.

Each of us is a unique individual with our own history, as well as simultaneously being the God Totality. God created the physical Universe in order to expand Itself through emotional experience and feeling. God is not a static state of being. It is the natural state of all beings to eternally expand in energetic consciousness and expression. Therefore, God is always expanding just as all Its incarnate soul expressions are eternally expanding both as individuals and as the totality. It is *emotional* embodiment that is the ingredient that allows for this expansion.

This is not to say that the mental body is inferior or should be rejected or ignored. Rather, we have over-focused on the mental body to avoid emotional experience, and it is a matter of integrating the emotional body into a balanced blend with the intellectual, physical and spiritual. The reason for centuries of imbalanced focus on intellectual learning is fear of the emotional body as well as the fearful denial of that fear.

We can read and learn and understand all we want so long as there is a genuine commitment to taking responsibility to own and feel the emotional experience and accept it as an equal aspect of our Selves. There is a tremendous amount of struggle and conflict taking place here because most of us stubbornly maintain the imbalance of the intellectual control over the emotional. This mental control, with its denial of the emotional body, is the foundation for all the struggle and conflict being experienced on Earth.

Emotional ownership means accepting who we are one hundred per cent as the creator of every moment and every detail of our lives. We are *not* victims of a victimizing universe, and nothing happens to us that has not been created on some level by us. We do not create some things in our lives and not others. We cannot be "a little bit pregnant." We either are or we aren't. In fact, we are pregnant with our eternally evolving spiritual Selves!

It is extremely important to understand that taking full responsibility for emotional ownership does *not* imply fault or blame. Most people define responsibility as assigning fault or blame. We say clearly that ownership means simply that and nothing more. Life is experience mirroring to us what we choose and create so that we can learn to make conscious choices and become who we want to be. The God Totality does not judge, blame, punish, reward or do anything that implies judgment.

Many people are afraid to "stick their toe into the water of emotional experience" because they project so much judgmental guilt, blame and expectations upon themselves and others. This pattern is part of the process that needs to be both owned and released in order to achieve true emotional ownership. As long as we judge or blame something, we are not owning or being who we are. As long as we project negative expectations, we are not being our Selves in the present moment. Emotional ownership means allowing us to see, feel and express whatever is going on in any moment and to do so without guilt, judgment, blame or expectation towards ourselves or others.

Nobody ever makes us feel or do anything. It is time to take our "mother made me . . .," and our "father made me . . ." statements and flush them down the toilet. Life will always reflect back in day-to-day experiences our issues that require our ownership and processing. In our dreams, we have our most direct dialogue with our Higher Selves in which we create symbols for the unresolved emotional issues whose healing will lead us to our spiritual expansion. Whatever is not resolved in the dream state is then projected, or (more accurately described as) solidified into our day-to-day life.

We magnetize to us individuals and events to act out these unresolved issues as another opportunity to own, feel and embody the unresolved issues that block our continued spiritual evolution. When we continue to deny and avoid the lessons and ownership in these daily-created experiences, the issues then solidify further to manifest in the physical body as illnesses and diseases.[5]

[5] Refer to Chapter 4 for this symbolic conversation of our bodies.

Many people fear the emotional process because they are afraid the emotions will hurt. We say, "Emotions are only emotions." It is not the emotions that create pain but rather the fearful resistance and denial of them. It is like learning to ice skate. If we are about to fall down and stiffen in fearful expectation, the fall may be very painful. If we just relax and fall, the pain will probably be much less if any at all. Learning that it is this mentally projected negative expectation of emotions that creates our pain rather than the emotions themselves is a major breakthrough to allow us to open up and feel our emotions with less drama and struggle.

Many people resist the emotional process because they are addicted to judging themselves and defining certain emotions as bad, evil, dark, unspiritual or disgusting. Any kind of judgment will certainly intensify the emotional experience. When we are willing to let go of judgmental definitions or negative expectations of emotions, a less painful and more graceful healing experience will unfold.

A stubborn, fearful mind does not want to give up its illusionary control and will hold on to defining and projecting negative judgments in order to keep the emotions away, convinced that it remains in control. This, of course, will lead to excessive drama, struggle and pain. Many of us are therefore addicted to acting like Drama Kings or Queens, to avoid the real emotions, convinced that nothing is real unless it is overly dramatic.

## Emotions & Emotional Ownership

It is important to be clear on the difference between emotions and feelings, especially since both are experienced the same way. Emotions are programmed reactions based on past-life experiences, whether or not we are conscious of it. It is important to be aware of our emotions to learn how we are subconsciously programmed to react to situations based on our life histories. This means we are not truly feeling and being who we are. When we become aware of what we emotionally feel in any situation and can see a pattern of repeating reactions, we can then begin to take conscious responsibility and control for what we choose to create and feel.

For example, if we share with someone a particular spiritual truth and they say, "You're crazy!" and we react by feeling hurt and stupid, it is important to be aware of this reaction and to let ourselves feel it. One of the most important keys is that everything we feel is real, but everything we feel is not necessarily true. So if we feel hurt or stupid because of a remark like that, it's a very real feeling.

After allowing ourselves to feel that emotion and see how we react, then it is important to ask, "What does this feeling tell me about myself?" If we choose to believe someone's projected judgment, some questions to ask are: Why do I choose to believe it? Do I not sufficiently trust my truth? Am I insecure with my truth to the point that I am addicted to validation or acceptance from others in order to feel safe?

Our emotional reactions help answer these questions. If we feel hurt or stupid because of the other person's judgmental statement, then this shows a lack of self-trust. Choose whether or not to feed more energy into the emotional reaction: Do I choose to remain feeling hurt? Do I choose to accept the feeling that I am stupid if someone else does not accept my truth? We are in control of our own lives. We are not victims unless we choose to victimize ourselves.

Here is another illustration: Let us say that your husband slaps you across the face when you serve him dinner. He says he hit you because dinner was late and tasteless and you're stupid and useless. What is your emotional reaction? Are you angry at his ignorant arrogance and lack of respect for you? Do you feel hurt, stupid, inferior and useless because you believe him? Do you feel that he is right and you are worthless unless you can do more and serve him "better"?

Here again, the emotional reaction reveals how we see ourselves and how we show ourselves to others. People treat us the way we perceive and treat ourselves. We magnetize people to interact with us as mirrors to reflect our self-perceptions. The next questions to ask are: Do we feel enough emotional reaction to no longer choose that kind of judging and hurtful experience and therefore choose to remove ourselves from any further experiences of that nature? Do we choose to feel like the "poor little victim" who needs to sacrifice and demean ourselves even more in order to get the acceptance that we do not feel worthy of? Do we buy into the experience or accept that this shows us something about our self-perception that we have the opportunity to heal and transform?

The abusive husband in the above example is one hundred per cent responsible for his emotional attack, even though his wife co-created the experience. The husband has chosen to play his role consciously or unconsciously because it is a role he wants to be in and/or has agreed to play out for his wife's learning experience. The wife has also consciously or unconsciously created her husband acting out this role for her own reasons. People who feel weak and inferior will choose to either act as a victim or as a victimizer, but the victim and victimizer are equal "victims" and are two sides of the same coin of self-rejection. Feeling our emotional reaction can lead us to this realization. It is important to not inject judgment, fault or guilt into it. The purpose is to act out our patterns so that we see what patterns are there, feel them one hundred per cent in order to derive all the learning experiences we can, and to then make a conscious creative choice of who we decide to be in each moment. Those who choose to act out the roles of victimizers do so from the same patterns of self-disgust, fear and denial as the victims. They repeatedly abuse the opportunity to take self-responsibility by attempting to escape feeling their self-disgust and self-judgment – maintaining an illusionary external control on their circumstances and upon other individuals.

Emotional ownership becomes total emotional healing when we have the discipline to ask ourselves in any situation: (1) What do I feel in this moment? (2) What does this feeling tell me about myself? (3) What do I choose to do with this? Remember to ask these questions again and again from one experience to another. This develops a conscious awareness and ownership of all emotional feelings and patterns which will, in turn, lead us to a more conscious healing and a more conscious choice in being who we want to be. Emotional Ownership means no longer being unconscious victims of external events from which an outside savior must rescue us.

It is precisely because emotional ownership removes the pattern of being a "helpless victim" needing to be "saved" by an outside savior that many choose to avoid or deny this ownership process. This is why people cling addictively to religious and New Age beliefs. Having the "right beliefs" will not save us. Believing in an external savior will not save us. Giving our emotions "to the light" will not heal anything. No guru will take away our karma or alleviate our emotional issues. We are our own creators, our creations and saviors. Christ Consciousness is not based on any religious belief system. It is not based on denying feelings and desires or "being less" on the Earth. Christ Consciousness is to feel and be one hundred per cent emotionally, mentally, spiritually and physically in the incarnate body here and now!

## Feelings vs. Emotions

Emotions are always reactions to memories and conditioning from the past. It is vital to recognize, feel and work through all the emotions to erase whatever behavior tapes are no longer lovingly constructive and supportive to us. It is also next to impossible to connect with our true feelings until we have recognized, owned, felt and processed all the emotional reactions *and* have done so without guilt, judgment, or negative expectations. Common examples of emotions are jealousy, envy, fear, hate, disgust and being in love (attraction to characteristics or qualities in others) as opposed to the spiritual feeling of love, which will be defined next.

Feelings are responses to being one hundred per cent in the present moment. When we experience true feelings, we are not subconsciously acting out a reactive history from other lifetime experiences. Rather, we are one hundred per cent present in the body in the moment as our total selves. Intuition is a feeling and is the most direct communication with the Higher Self. Even if we hear a voice with intuition, it is nevertheless experienced as a feeling from our innermost depths.

Whereas the emotion "in-love" involves attractions based on needs and history, the feeling love is an acceptance and embodiment that is not based on need, fear or expectation. It is a sense of total acceptance and being that contains no sense of incompletion or inadequacy. Whereas the emotion of sympathy involves personal attachment or identification, the feeling of empathy allows for an unconditional compassion and understanding of another's experience that does not require personal involvement. Other feelings such as joy and bliss are not about denial of any desires or needs — which they are often misrepresented as — but are rather unconditional acceptance of total beingness.

Emotions are always conditional because they are based on reactions (whether consciously or unconsciously) and on a sense of insecurity or inadequacy. Feelings are always an unconditional acceptance of being. The more we accept individuals and experiences in our everyday lives as opportunities to feel and learn these differences, the greater the potential for healing and expansion. The book *A Course in Miracles* has as one of its daily lessons, "I am never upset for the reason I think." This is an excellent lesson to keep in mind when approaching the process of emotional ownership. What makes life more painful and chaotic is our subconscious reaction rather than the emotion itself. When we are willing to experience any moment without judging or needing expected results, this relaxing and accepting into the moment can alleviate much of the suffering and struggle.

The more we try to avoid or escape something, the more we cause it and become it. Whatsoever we love the most in anyone or anything, the more that mirrors the same quality in us that perhaps is not yet fully felt and recognized. The more we hate anything in someone else, the more we tend to deny and avoid that quality within ourselves. We choose and create every moment based on what will most assist us to heal and grow. We need to accept this without guilt, blame, fault or judgment. The more we are willing to trust that whatever we feel reveals something we are ready to experience, embody, feel and heal, the easier the process can be and the greater the healing.

# Chapter 4
# Body Symbology & Taking Personal Responsibility

Taking personal responsibility for our lives means noting our patterns and emotions, and how we drew them all to ourselves. There is no one to blame for anything. If we don't like what is in our lives, the place to start is always within ourselves.

It is important to develop a personal honor code that states the ground rules for how we choose to relate to ourselves and to others as well as how we choose for others to treat us. If we constantly meet people who do not love, accept or respect us, we have the opportunity to learn to love, accept and respect ourselves. Each person is there to mirror an aspect of us.

## Body Symptoms

Before discussing the specific examples of symbology in diseases and body parts, it is important to understand that there are people who experience few or no symptoms in their bodies as well as those who experience an abundance of body symptoms.

Some people assume that if nothing bad is happening in their bodies, this must indicate they are highly evolved with little or no issues. Not necessarily so! Those who don't have many physical symptoms going on in their bodies may be in one of two categories: (1) They may have simply chosen to learn their lessons in another format. (2) Some people have established such a powerful denial defense that it keeps the body shut down from expressing symbolic messages. This can eventually lead to a major crisis in the body and/or the external life experience. Only in extremely rare cases is perfect or near perfect health a direct manifestation of the health of the soul. We're talking here about individuals such as Yeshua Ben Yosef (Jesus), Siddharta Gautama (Buddha) or St. Germain.

People may panic from an assumption that if things begin to happen in their bodies as they become more consciously committed to their spiritual paths, then something is wrong. For example, when we begin to channel messages from alternate levels of consciousness (whether through automatic writing, trance-channeling or spontaneous conscious channeling), we will often experience periods of headaches, insomnia, increase in mucus, diarrhea or flu-like symptoms.

The same is true with a person who has made an increased devotion to their spiritual and healing pathway on the planet. These are not automatically signs that they are ill or that something is wrong. On the contrary, the body is triggering a massive cleansing of physical toxins in response to the higher frequencies of energy being introduced into the aura and the physical body. We specifically discuss this topic at the end of this chapter. Refer to "Physical Symptoms to Watch for upon Making Spiritual Changes."

Any increase in energy or consciousness accelerates the vibrations of the emotional body. Denied emotions manifest as physical toxins and energy blockages. Any healing or releasing of emotional suppression will immediately trigger a purging of physical toxins or blockages. Keeping this in mind can assist us in a natural healing process rather than panicking and attacking a healing process as if it were a negative problem. We will address this topic again in more detail after we go through the body symbology.

## "Soul Tourists"

Some souls are on what we call a "tourist incarnation" in which they are allowed a lifetime to rest from a previously traumatic incarnation. This is like taking a vacation to Hawaii to unwind from all the stress in our third dimensional lives. When our vacation is over, we go back to our "other" life.

A "tourist life" is not an automatic statement of "high" or "low" spiritual development. It is simply that a soul is sometimes allowed a "rest" life to integrate previous experiences so as to more efficiently proceed on its path later in this life or in the next incarnation. Be careful not to judge these souls as lazy or "not doing anything." You may have just come from a "tourist" incarnation, which is why you have such a "get up and go" attitude in this lifetime!

## Body Symbology

Our Higher Selves communicate with us in our dreams, relaying messages about our unresolved issues. What isn't worked out at the dream level is then moved into the externalized third-dimensional life. If we continue to resist or deny the issues on that level, it next manifests in the body. The body communicates with us all the time, telling us what is building up in our cellular structure and our energetic integrity. We either listen or we don't.

Diseases occur because emotional denials are projected and acted out into our third dimensional lives. Most people tend to focus on *how* they got sick rather than *why*. Allopathic Medicine focuses on the "how" while spirituality focuses on the "why." It is time for these two areas to come together. In true self-healing it is important to go beyond the symptoms of "how" and feel the true emotional issues that, with continued suppression and denial, build up energetically to create the disease or disorder in the body.

It is important to understand how and why we magnetize certain things to us. If it were true that viruses, germs, bacteria or pollution were *all* there were to disease, then all of us would be sick all the time. We are constantly bombarded by billions of factors, yet they don't always cause disease. Illness occurs because our consciousness magnetizes to us an experience of what we own or don't own or what we accept or resist in our emotional process.

## How the Body Communicates with Us

Different parts of the body resonate particular symbolic messages about our emotional denials that are seeking recognition, feeling, acceptance, and healing. Aches and pains generally suggest fearful and stubborn resistance. The *location* of pain in the body can offer more specific information about characteristics within us that are calling for closer attention from us. Cancer and other diseases may illustrate issues about self-hatred. The particular location of the cancer or other types of disease can give more specific details about the how, where and what of the issue being communicated by the body.

Thoughts and emotions are magnetically creative energies. People who hold on to mental beliefs that are very limiting, self-denying and self-rejecting will magnetize "accidents" in which they get concussions, dislocate shoulders, acquire sprains, or break bones (such as hands and wrists.) The hands can say to us, "I can't handle this." When we stubbornly hold on to self-limiting thoughts or feelings, these energies become crystallized toxins in the body. They will go to whatever part of the body represents the issue we are working out. For example, when it is a mental addiction that we stubbornly hold onto and we feel, "I can't handle this," we can create injuries or infections to the hands, arms or shoulders. This is a signal that we fear to embrace or handle something that needs to be owned, accepted and felt.

How and where a certain emotional issue expresses itself in a person's body depends on the mental, emotional and spiritual issues involved in each case. For example, both asthma and diabetes are *emotionally* caused by suppressed feelings of being unlovable. The reason why one emotional issue can manifest as two such different diseases is that they are part of different emotional-mental-spiritual complexes. With asthma, there is an accompanying sense of worthlessness to the extreme of not even feeling worthy to draw breath. With diabetes, one feels unlovable because of fearing the power and responsibility that comes with being loved.

When engaging in self-healing, remember that all ailments of the body are one hundred percent *caused* by suppressed emotions. The *reason* why the emotions are blocked and suppressed is one hundred percent because of mental self-judgments, denials, and lack of self-love. And the *mechanisms* through which the diseases manifest themselves in our bodies are one hundred percent physical. One of the major differences between East and West is that we in the West like to think in absolutes, while the people of the East think in terms of paradoxes and apparent contradictions much more easily than we do. When we (the authors) tell people about the emotional component of an illness, they often respond with something such as, "No, it's not emotional, it's an infection. There is something physically there!"

It's very hard for people trained in the Western way of thinking to understand that it's not a matter of either/or. Diseases do not have either a physical cause or an emotional cause. It's both. And it's not even half-physical and half-emotional. It's simultaneously one hundred percent physical and one hundred percent emotional. In addition, it's also one hundred percent mental. An Eastern mind would have no problem grasping this, while a typical Western mind would immediately start adding the percentages up and get an impossible 300% of causes. The *mechanics* of all diseases are always one hundred percent physical. The *cause* is always one hundred percent emotional. The *reason* is always one hundred percent mental and spiritual.

Here's a classic example from physics to serve as an illustration. In science, we can study light either as a wave or as a particle, never as both. We have to observe it as one or the other. We observe it as a wave, and then only as a wave, one hundred percent, or we observe it as a particle, and then only as a particle, again one hundred percent. Thus, anyone who remembers their physics from high school can easily see that light is simultaneously one hundred percent a wave and one hundred percent a particle.

It is the same with our physical bodies and their ailments. We can look at all diseases from a purely physical point of view. Or we can look at the psychosomatic element of every disease. But the truth is that it is never a matter of either physical, emotional or mental. Nor is it ever part physical and part emotional or mental. It is always all three of them one hundred percent each.

Another reason why people fail to see the emotional component of their illness, and even expend a lot of energy in maintaining their denial of it, is that it is in the nature of suppressed emotions to be relegated to our subconscious. So of course we're not aware of the suppressed emotion… until it manifests as a disease in our bodies. The fact that the denied emotions are subconscious is the very reason why they make our bodies become sick. They make our bodies sick in order to make the denials in our subconscious heard and noticed by our conscious awareness. What a gift!

Ironically enough, the fact that these denied emotions are subconscious and have to go to such drastic measures to be noticed by us is also the reason why we often deny the emotional cause of our diseases. We've never been consciously aware of "that particular emotion," so we can't see how an emotion we're not aware of having could possibly be the cause of our physical ailment, especially since we "know for a fact" that it's caused by a bacteria or whatever physical element.

Do you see the dilemma that our emotions and bodies are in? This process of listening to what our bodies communicate to us about what is stored in our subconscious takes practice. It can be very enjoyable and fulfilling once we learn that it's not a matter of looking through our inner recesses for "bad things" to purge ourselves of.

Try not to judge or condemn your previously suppressed emotions when you discover that you have them because that judgement is exactly what made them hide away in your subconscious to begin with! Instead, treat them as you would a frightened child. Take them in your arms and hold them there, lovingly, warm and safe, until all their fear has dissipated. Allow them to express everything they need to express, their sounds coming through your throat and their movements expressing through your body. That is how you can heal your so-called "negative" emotions.

## The Astrological Body Symbols

We include astrology in this book because it is a form of symbolic language at a higher level of consciousness, just as dreams are a symbolic language between the conscious incarnate soul and the Higher Self. We feel that the astrological signs, the karmic lesson(s) and body part they represent are important aspects to go along with the fact that parts of the body and diseases are symbolic messages of denied emotional and spiritual patterns manifesting in physical form.

Some people may believe or disbelieve in astrology for the wrong reasons. Planets and their movements do not determine our lives. Rather, they are used to portray symbolic qualities and energy forces projected to us by a consciously alive Universe.

Astrology does not tell us what will happen or what we must do. The Cosmos reflects karmic patterns and energetic tendencies created by individual and mass human consciousness in a symbolic form to catalyze and challenge us to higher awareness and deeper inner-attunement and self-ownership.

As a general introduction to body symbology, we list the twelve signs of the zodiac, the karmic lessons they represent, and the part of the body corresponding to the astrological sign:

| Astrological Sign | Karmic Lesson | Body Part |
|---|---|---|
| Aries | I Am | Head |
| Taurus | I Have | Neck |
| Gemini | I Think | Shoulders, Arms, Hands, Lungs |
| Cancer | I Feel | Breasts, Stomach |
| Leo | I Will | Heart, Spine |
| Virgo | I Analyze, I Perfect | Intestines, Liver, Bladder, Gall - Bladder, Pancreas |
| Libra | I Balance | Kidneys, Skin, Lymphatic System, Blood |
| Scorpio | I Desire | Sexual Organs, Prostate |
| Sagittarius | I See | Hips, Thighs |
| Capricorn | I Use | Knees, Skeleton |
| Aquarius | I Know | Shins, Calves |
| Pisces | I Become, I Integrate, I Transform | Feet |

To illustrate how to use the above chart, suppose that you suffer from arthritis in the hands and want to know the deeper message behind the arthritic symptoms. Looking on the chart you see the hands are under the category of Gemini, whose karmic lesson is, "I Think." What are you thinking that is causing some kind of stress or resistance in your life? As you will see further in this chapter, arthritis is a manifestation of stubborn resistance. Arthritis in the hands, represented by Gemini, indicates that it is a stubborn resistance in your thinking that causes you to not "handle" something in your life that needs a deeper intuitive recognition.

If arthritis manifests in the knees, which are under the category of Capricorn with its karmic lesson "I Use," the stubbornness message of the arthritis here indicates how you use or act out resistance, causing stress to the body. Many people will have arthritis in all or many joints simultaneously because the body symbolizes the interaction of stress and difficulties caused by the stubborn thinking process and how it expresses itself through various daily actions and usage. So the body clearly illustrates how thought causes action which thereby results in the arthritic manifestation.

## Examples of Symbolic Body Communications

The information which follows is a partial list to give examples on how the body communicates symbolically to reveal the physical consequences of mental and/or emotional fear, resistance and denial. We didn't list all disease conditions at this point. Perhaps we will do that in another book.

These physical symptoms are also created to illustrate that we can re-create any situation to whatever we truly desire as well as to prove that we have the power to balance and heal anything through our willingness to open up to self-love and self-responsibility without guilt or judgment.

No matter how painful or horrible something may feel or appear to be, every experience is a positive opportunity to choose to use power to heal rather than to engage in self-denial and self-destruction. It takes enormous strength to feel weak, and any disorder or dysfunction is an opportunity to meet that strength and choose to be strong and healed.

Please note that these are generalizations to get you started. It is important to read each section that pertains to you and to think/feel/perceive if it is true for you *in this moment*. We are merely giving you a start. It is up to you to dive deeper into yourself to discover the message your Higher Self feels is important to communicate.

Also remember that you may have fallen and broken your ankle when you were five years old, which had a particular meaning and message in your life at that time. Now at age 74 if you fall and break your ankle again, it may have a different message for you. There are no absolutes, and no one outside of you can give you the meaning of what happens to you. It is simply our intention to make your inner exploration more enjoyable with this book and to provide a few clues along the way. The rest is up to you! It is our heartfelt wish that you en-*Joy* your journey!

We will now list the conditions according to regions in the body, proceeding from the Head to the Feet. Some listings could go under several categories. For instance, Arthritis is a degenerative condition. However, we listed it under *Skeleton, Spine & Joints* as we felt more people would look there. So, look around this chapter if you don't find what you are looking for in the place you expected to find it.

# The Nervous System

## Neurological Disorders

The brain, spinal cord and nerves throughout the body (peripheral nerves) together comprise what is generally called neurological tissue. This tissue is responsible for sending and receiving billions of communications. These are the communications that keep the entire body functioning as a unit. If a few nerve cells or a certain nerve is damaged, perhaps other cells or nerves can carry the same impulse, and the body adapts. However, when larger portions of this neurological tissue lose its functioning power, we lose certain abilities. These can include speech, hearing, muscle movement, mental abilities, and the functioning of organs or glands associated with the nerve tissue involved. Some of the names medical scientists give to these losses of functions in the nervous system include Alzheimer's, Lou Gehrig's (ALS), Multiple Sclerosis (MS), Parkinson's, Huntington's Chorea and others.

In general, our neurological system symbolizes how we communicate with our own inner energies. When this inner communication flows freely, our level of integrity — how we see and honor our own inner truths — can be mirrored to us through our neurological system. When we are out of harmony with our own inner truths, we create inflammation, which represents self-anger. We create nerve paralysis when we have so much fear residing in us that we can't take any action. We can lose certain other body functions when we don't listen or communicate to portions of our bodies via our nerve pathways.

It is important to feel into this area for each person, because neurological challenges may represent a lack of willingness to communicate with others. If a person is experiencing so much fear and lack of trust within themselves, they are hesitant to communicate to others. Thus, they may get symptoms of nerve pathways not working properly producing symptoms such as jerking of muscles, tingling and numbness of the hands, arms or legs.

## Alzheimer's Disease

Alzheimer's disease is a manifestation of a soul's lack of desire to remain in a physical body. Most often those who have been highly dependent upon their intellectual skills as a source of personal identity and self-value meet one or several crises that call for a level of emotional ownership and expression that is too terrifying for that person to experience. There is a panic about continuing their life as their dependency on their intellectual capabilities is not sufficient to meet the emotional crisis or crises arising in their lives.

A manifestation such as Alzheimer's will express in the body as the soul attempts to escape physical reality. Yet simultaneously, the soul is terrified to "pass over" into the etheric realm of existence where they will still have to face and process the issue they are trying to escape from in the physical incarnation. Trapped in a kind of limbo world between terror to live and terror to pass on with no sense of foundation or protection from their intellectual skills, these souls linger in an experience of deterioration until the body tires of the energetically exhausting struggle and surrenders the tie of the soul to the physical realm. Alzheimer's is an opportunity for the soul to recognize the over-dependency upon intellectualism and how it denies and cuts off the emotional body, so that the soul may eventually allow itself to be open to the opportunities of nurturing, healing love, and learning experiences awaiting its willingness to open up to its emotional experiences.

## Anxiety/Panic Attacks

Like Obsessive Compulsive Disorder, anxiety or panic attacks stem from a rush of emotions coming to the surface. They are generally stimulated by something that is stressful, such as being in a small, enclosed space (an elevator, for instance), being in a crowded room, or being in a car during rush hour traffic.

During an anxiety attack, the space seems to close in on the person. They experience intense fear and may have difficulty breathing, may feel they are going to have a heart attack or some other serious health challenge.

What helps during these attacks is to first of all breathe deeply. Allow your emotions to surface and express them however it seems the most appropriate. Don't edit yourself! In other words, cry, scream, or allow whatever happens to be all right. If you have some calming essential oils, you can use those. However, don't do it with the intention of suppressing your emotions. If the essential oils help to regulate the flow of the anxiety attack, then use them to give you some sense of control.

Yes, there are physical supplements one can take which change the way the neurotransmitters (brain chemicals) work at the synapses in the brain. However, this is only on the physical level. These won't change the emotions one needs to move which may have been repressed for many lifetimes.

## Crippling

Sometimes souls choose a "crippling" experience to teach themselves that they have the power within them to overcome any limitation and not be crippled in their true spiritual being by any external conditions or situations. Often this is also an experience to teach those around the soul that they can overcome and transmute anything.

## Numbness/Paralysis

When portions of our bodies become numb or paralyzed, this is a major signal from our bodies that we are unconscious in some way, or that we block the communication from our Higher Selves or Inner God Selves. We are not fully present in life for whatever reason. The important part in our healing is to discover where we sent our energies, what it is we choose not to address or pay attention to, or why we punish ourselves by creating parts of our bodies no longer working in an optimal manner.

There are always positive reasons why certain traumatic events happen to us. In certain cases, we choose to shut down certain body parts because this allows us to discover different ways of working with our bodies. Another reason for shut down is to enable us to experience emotions that we wouldn't otherwise have allowed ourselves to feel. It is self-sabotaging and judgmental to think that we are always only punishing ourselves with an illness or incapacity.

## Obsessive Compulsive Disorder (OCD)

There is an increasing awareness of Obsessive Compulsive Disorder (OCD) in our society today. This is due not only to heightened understanding and media coverage, but also to a very real increase of this pattern in the human souls currently on Earth. Repressed emotional memories are being driven upwards from the cellular level into conscious human awareness and behavior.

OCD is the result of an ongoing sense of unsafety that souls increasingly feel from incarnation to incarnation as their suppressed, denied emotions are forced to the conscious surface by the natural spiraling intensity of cosmic evolution. It is becoming harder and harder to suppress and deny our emotions, and this is stimulating a severe panic in many human souls who fear self-ownership and responsibility and who try to remain hidden beneath the addiction to belief systems, judgments, religious rituals and an external God/Savior. OCD is used to cover up the terror of this panic and the unsafety of being incarnated at this time.

Compulsive actions result from obsessive thoughts, and the obsessive thoughts derive from the suppressed emotional memories, guilt and self-judgment of past-life choices and behavior. The compulsive behavior to lock a door, turn off an appliance or check a dozen times or more to be sure it has been done, stems from the obsessive thought that something has not been completed or not completed correctly or adequately. The foundation of OCD patterns is often a self-judgmental fear that in a past life some choice or responsibility was not done at the right time or in the right way. This then resulted in someone else being injured, blamed, killed, etc. The gnawing guilt and self-judgments are so deep and relentless as to become unbearable to the soul's memory. It is then suppressed under the OCD pattern so that as the emotion continues to be denied, it is replaced by the obsessive thought and compulsive behavior. Nothing will ever be final or good enough so long as this judgment-filled guilt remains suppressed and denied beneath the OCD pattern.

A person who needs to constantly wash and re-wash their hands, bodies, clothes or home, or who has an obsessive fear of germs have a deeply suppressed judgment of some past-life actions(s) being "dirty" and making the soul spiritually "unclean" or "disgusting."

In all cases of OCD patterns, healing involves letting go of judgment and guilt, releasing the concept that nothing they do is ever good enough and then allowing themselves to feel the underlying emotions that are covered up by the disorder. There are many psychological therapies and support groups for OCD. Psychodrama, voice-dialogue therapy and the use of Gem Elixirs, Flower Essences and essential oils may be able to assist in bringing the suppressed emotional memory, fear, judgment or guilt to the surface where it can be recognized, accepted and released. Practitioners of Vibrational Medicine and essential oils can tune in to particular essences or combinations that can assist individuals in the healing of OCD patterns.

## Tremors

A tremor is a condition in which the muscles produce alternating contractions. There are tremors that occur at any time (involuntary), and those that only occur when movement is initiated (intention tremor). Tremors, like convulsions, occur to "jump start" or awaken the body and one's consciousness. They are often signals from the body that messages or feelings are trying to get through that are being denied and suppressed, consciously or subconsciously, by the incarnate soul.

# Addictions

We have become a nation of addicts. Whether it is alcohol, drugs, sugar, caffeine, tobacco, gambling, sex, shopping, or food, we all search for balance. Addictions are a signal to us that it is time to make changes, that our bodies are malnourished and our Spirits are broken. Our addictions teach us that we are denying ourselves emotional healing and nurturing, which we cover up in self-destructive behavior. Until we answer the body's call for deeper emotional commitment to ourselves and until we stop feeling the need to punish ourselves, our addictive behavior will continue its erosion of the body, mind and soul.

One of the most powerful addictions is the addiction to belief systems. Religious fundamentalists identify themselves with their beliefs to the point of being threatened by anything not of their belief system and to the point of being cut off from true heart-feeling. The more they talk about love, the more heartless they act.

Another imprisoning heart addiction is how we identify ourselves with our diseases and patterns: "I am an alcoholic," "I am an abuse survivor," "I am a diabetic," "I am arthritic," "I am a victim of cancer." We become so *identified* with what is going on in our bodies that we make it extremely difficult to heal or move on to what is next for us.

Even when we desperately want to be healed and pain-free, the *identification* to what is going on in the body is such a powerfully addictive prison that we can actually be threatened by the reality of being healed without consciously realizing it. To be free of pain or a disease becomes, on a deep unconscious level, a threat to our identity and existence, even as we simultaneously desire to be healed. This paradox is very difficult for many people to realize and own, thereby strengthening the stranglehold of the addictive belief or the addictive sense of identity.

The need to judge or punish ourselves for choices, actions or health conditions is an addiction that only intensifies and prolongs painful experiences. It is far more loving and healing to accept responsibility for choices and actions without the need to condemn or punish oneself. Otherwise, this addictive perspective leads to repeatedly painful experiences, even when a lesson has already been acknowledged.

Addiction is a call to develop a truly loving relationship to oneself. We seek to give to ourselves, and we don't know how, so we "give" ourselves alcohol and other drugs in a feeble attempt at self-nurturing. When we can really learn to listen to our inner voice, stop judging and condemning ourselves and learn to give self-love, then we will stop wanting to drink, drug or eat ourselves into oblivion. There are many emotional patterns that want to come to the surface to be acknowledged and addressed in addiction.

Addiction is all about covering up shame, pain, sadness and sorrow, easing guilt, and even punishing the self for one's perceived wrong-doings. Again, we choose to cover up something because we judge it as being something that is wrong with us. When we can look at this as our soul's attempt to create an opening for healing, we can celebrate our addictive patterns by dropping our judgments and thus bring these patterns to their natural completion.

## Alcoholism

Alcoholism is the great disease of spirituality. Souls choose alcoholism when they are most desperate for a spiritual opening from rigid boundaries. Alcoholism is a way to blast one's boundaries — to experience a pattern in the extreme. It is a breakthrough from self-condemnation.

It is no coincidence that we refer to alcohol as "spirits." Alcoholism is a cry for spirituality distorted into an addictive behavior due to self-judgmental condemnation that tries to convince us we are not truly worthy of what we desire. It is an opportunity to overcome an inner crisis and reveal to us that we can use our power equally to heal and transform as well as to condemn and destroy.

It is impossible to measure the support, healing love and overwhelming impact Alcoholics Anonymous has had on hundreds of thousands of peoples' lives. One must celebrate with the highest respect and appreciation the tireless guidance and support this organization has given to so many. But we also want to say to Alcoholics Anonymous to please be willing to accept the reality that they do not live in a universe where any disease is incurable. To stand up before others and say "I am an alcoholic" takes tremendous courage and commitment to self-responsibility and healing. It confronts the soul with the pattern of denial and offers the opportunity to free oneself of endless blind denial and begin a path to healing. But to endlessly need to say "I am an alcoholic" year after year — and to be told that alcoholism is an incurable disease — causes a soul to identify itself so profoundly with the disease as to make it almost impossible to be free of it. It then becomes threatening for the subconscious to accept a reality where the alcoholism is fully healed because the identity of the disease and one's self become fused. To believe that a disease is incurable is an addictive belief. To accept that alcoholism is incurable is to exchange one addiction for another.

Likewise, much energy is being put into the belief, "I am an alcoholic (or any other addiction or disease) because it is in my genes." Yes, it *is* in your genes. But it is in your genes because your genetic code is a physical manifestation of your accumulated[6] emotions, thoughts, beliefs and expectations. Being in our genes can answer the question of *how* we act out a pattern, but it does not answer *why*. The why is in the history of the emotional body and in the beliefs one chooses to accept.

It is vitally important to remember that nothing of this is a matter of blame or fault. We choose and create (consciously or unconsciously) from the accumulative history of what we choose to feel, think and accept as truth. The purpose of alcoholism or any addiction or disease is to illustrate this to us through our consciously or unconsciously creative life experiences.

Saying "I am an alcoholic" *for a period of time* helps to clear denial and accept self-responsibility, especially when one can do so *without* the addictive need for guilt, blame, fault, self-condemnation or punishment. But there needs to come a time when it is no longer necessary to say "I am an alcoholic" or else it can become an addictive brainwashing. *All* diseases are curable. There is no such thing in this universe as an incurable disease. To believe anything is incurable is to trap oneself in *another* addiction.

## Drug Addiction

The rampant drug addiction on this planet is a reflection of mixed messages. On the one hand, souls use drugs to suppress emotions and memories too painful or frightening to

[6] From this and all previous lifetimes.

feel. There is an attempt to escape what they do not trust they can handle. At the same time, these souls are symbolically acting out an attempt to heal their inner torments. Western medicine has brainwashed us into believing that the prime directive is to take a pill to get rid of physical symptoms. Hence, souls in crisis act out their addictive behavior to solve or escape problems through drug usage. Acceptance, support and training to recognize, feel, honor and learn from emotional feelings and signals is vital to alleviating this ever-consuming addictive behavior.

## Enabler/Over Care-Taker

Oftentimes we focus on addictions which go through our mouth (or other orifices) such as alcohol, cigarettes, drugs to swallow, shoot or inhale. Some of the most difficult addictions to identify and heal are those patterns of being the victim, the martyr and especially the over care-taker. In these addictions, we feed off another's pain or dysfunction and we get our "fix" by them continuing in their imbalance. Many times when the addict is in recovery or has been clean/sober a period of time, the enabler or over care-taker leaves the person to seek another source for their addiction.

In healing this type of addiction, it is imperative that the over care-taker seek an identity and a life purpose related to themself, rather than through another person. It is important to stop running away from the self through taking care of another, and attune to one's own healing.

## Food Addiction

We suppress our deepest emotional memories, fears and denials in the solar plexus. This is why addiction to food is so prevalent in emotionally unhappy individuals. On the one hand, we use food in an attempt to further bury those denied emotional feelings, while at the same time eating and eating to try and fill the void of self-rejection with physical nourishment to replace the absence of emotional and spiritual nourishment. No matter what or how much we eat, the fullness and satisfaction will not be achieved. Food cannot compensate for the real emotional ownership and experience that the body and soul need.

### Sex Addiction

An addiction to sex can be caused by a soul who has been caught up in very religious lifetimes of sexual fear, judgment or denial, such as former monks and nuns. Religion is a human-made invention for control, caused by fear of power. When we are ready to own our power, we must let go of the judgmental fear and denial, otherwise the pendulum sways to the extreme opposite. It achieves an equilibrium when the individual integrates by experiencing all aspects of power and sexuality.

## Head

The head symbolizes how we perceive or define ourselves as individuals and how we choose to express that definition of ourselves to the outside world. It is a very common pattern, for example, for people who have been very emotionally and/or spiritually "asleep" to create a traumatic head injury, brain aneurysm or a brain tumor in order to manifest a life opportunity to consciously awaken to deeper inner potentials. When the body feels there is too much intellectual energy over-controlling and suppressing the emotional body, some kind of brain trauma can occur to awaken the soul to "get out of the head," to provide a greater balance with the rest of the body. Then that person's spiritual journey can more profoundly "take off" after such an injury. The message here is, "I need to wake up and get on with it."

## Acne

There are primarily two reasons why a soul chooses to create acne in the face. One is that we have subconscious feelings of being "dirty" and disgusting, which are not consciously felt and acknowledged. So the body manifests acne to force us to feel these feelings of self-disgust that we are attempting to suppress and deny.

Another common reason for creating acne is that we are unconsciously afraid of the attention we would get if we looked more attractive. So we create acne to protect ourselves from too much sexual or romantic attention. At the same time, there is almost certainly another part of us that longs to be more attractive and have more attention. In that way, acne also serves to bring to our attention an internal conflict that we were probably not aware of.

## Blindness

Blindness contains the obvious symbol of people who don't want to see that physical reality is a mirror of internal creative choices. People don't want to see what they don't want to take ownership for in themselves. Sometimes people choose blindness because physical incarnation is so terrifying and threatening. It is an attempt to sever groundedness in physical experience.

Blindness can also be chosen as a way to train a soul to be more attuned to their intuition and focus on the inner spiritual/psychic sight and not be distracted by the external world that they may have escaped into in past lives to avoid that deep attunement to their intuitive gifts.

## Brain Tumors

Refer to Cysts & Tumors under Degenerative Conditions on page 138.

## Cataracts

Cataracts symbolize specific "blind spots" people attempt to set up in their lives to avoid owning whatever life issues they do not feel safe to see and work with. Cataracts reflect a selective sight people choose to use as an excuse to not see their own resistant denials.

## Deafness

Deafness can be a severe rejection of a lesson or responsibility a soul doesn't want to hear. Sometimes deafness is also created by the Higher Self to force people who get caught up with hearing too much around them to force them deeper inside themselves so that they can learn to listen with their heart and soul and not be preoccupied by external stimuli. They need to focus upon and be more developed to inner intuitive listening.

## Dyslexia

Dyslexia is actually a hearing disorder caused by a dysfunction in the brain that results in an individual being right ear dominant instead of left ear dominant. This may be confusing to people who will say, "But I'm not listening to anything when I'm trying to read and the letters are transposed." We don't have to be hearing anything at the moment to experience the dyslexia. The very fact that we have created ourselves to be right ear dominant causes the messages in the brain to be switched. Souls create this condition because they are trying to mix up the messages in their brains so as to not hear or see clearly what they need to heal and resolve in this lifetime. Especially souls who have experienced several lifetimes of abusive physical beatings have built up such a sense of inferiority and inadequacy that they feel they are not capable of normal learning and understanding. They then switch the dominance from left ear to right ear so that all the signals in the brain flow in the opposite direction.

Dyslexia can be healed by training the individual to listen more intently through the left ear. This can be done, for example, by wearing earphones and listening to music or words in which for long periods of time the right earphone is turned off. This helps stimulate the left ear to listen more which will then start the energy signals to flow left to right rather than right to left. When one works with oneself to listen more through the left ear, this balancing will then result in the visually dyslexic condition reversing itself so that reading can be achieved properly.

Dyslexia is a manifestation of feeling a severe inadequacy due to past-life physical abuse trauma. Usually this is not sexual abuse, which tends to appear in other parts of the body. Dyslexia is a manifestation of physical beating, especially people who have been beaten often on the ears and around the head. The severe feelings of inadequacy and stupidity that are derived from such prolonged physical beatings need proper emotional clearing through whatever therapies are best for the individual. This, combined with training the person to listen more with the left ear, can result in a one hundred per cent healing of the dyslexic condition.

## Glaucoma

Glaucoma is an intense fear of death or major life changes which the individual is too threatened to surrender to and experience. It is an attempt to "fog" the issue so as to procrastinate the inevitable they are trying to keep at bay as long as possible because they do not trust that they are ready, or adequate to face it. Whereas cataracts mirror very specific blind spots someone puts up in front of them to create temporary obstacles, glaucoma is a more intense overall panic in which they are trying to cover up everything. Ninety-nine per cent of the time, glaucoma communicates the fear of old age and death and the inevitability of one's life cycle.

## Hair

Hair is an archetype of strength and courage. There is Samson's story in the Bible in which his hair was cut off, resulting in a lack of strength. Problems with losing hair or scalp are also due to a lack of emotional trust and the feeling of a lack of emotional and physical support in life. Male-pattern baldness often results from suppressed guilt towards past-life experiences of abusing masculine power by overly aggressive behavior or by addictive control over others.

## Headaches

Headaches are one of the most common afflictions of the human race with the underlying causes as numerous and varied as the people affected. There are many physical reasons for headaches: migraines, tension, toxins in the system, structural misalignment, a lack of oxygen, a lack of proper hydration, digestive and blood sugar related. Headaches can also be caused by changes in the weather, worms or parasites in the brain.

The brain becomes dehydrated after drinking alcohol or caffeine, which causes more water to leave the body than one is taking in. Oxygen delivery is impaired when the blood vessels are congested and also when the muscles in the neck and head are tight, or in spasm. The brain uses more oxygen and blood sugar than any other part of the body, so it is important to make sure it gets its needs met.

Migraine headaches are more severe and on a physical level, they may have their origin in the intestines. Migraines also occur in the presence of too much estrogen, or the lack of sufficient progesterone. On an emotional level, migraine headaches can occur in people working through their fears who exhibit heavy control issues. Because migraines occur on only one side of the head, they can represent a conflict between one's masculine and feminine energies. Another group of people that commonly suffer from migraines are those who are extremely emotional, but who simultaneously are in severe judgment of their own emotionality.

Some cases of headaches occur in people who are overly dependent on their intellectual capacity, using their mental body as an overcompensation for their lack of stimulation (and lack of trust) in their emotional body. With people who are too much in their head, their aura can emanate out from the head area 10-30 feet. Then from the shoulders on down, the aura can shrink down to as little as 1/8 inch! The aura can radiate partially beside them rather than appropriately around them, or they can be dragging it behind them like a shadow when not one hundred percent centered in the body emotionally as well as mentally and physically.

There is no one definition of how far an aura should radiate. Rather, the emanation should be equal around the whole body. It is not automatically true that we are more enlightened because our aura extends thirty feet away from our physical bodies. Nor do we need to pull in our auras, thinking that to touch another's aura is in any way bad. Our auras penetrate one another as a way of triggering the mirroring and support we give to one another. The most important issue is the equalized balance of the aura surrounding the body.

## Teeth & Gums

Loose teeth, teeth rotting or falling out, or problems with the gums serve as a symbol to illustrate a lack of trust in one's emotional strength and courage. They symbolize something we don't feel safe to work with.

On a physical level, someone who has an unhealthy diet, who eats too much sugar or extremely spicy food, does so as an overcompensation because of a long-standing pattern with these issues involving denial of self-love and self-trust. Thus, damage to the teeth as a result of diet and the emotional compensation in one's eating habits merge into a unified symbolic message of this denial of inner courage and trust.

# Neck

We put into our necks all the daily frustrations and fears about not having enough to meet our needs. When we over-identify ourselves with what we have or don't have, (or what we value or don't value), that consciousness goes into the neck.

When we fear we don't have enough to physically take care of ourselves, this creates frustrated energy that becomes a hard blockage in the neck. Crystallized toxins wrap around the vertebrae and nerve cords in the neck. This results in a stiff neck or other neck pain, and the lymph glands become blocked with crystallized toxins from these kinds of thoughts.

We also get sore throats, throat infections and laryngitis which shows up in this region of the body. These conditions generally occur when we are not expressing our inner truth, or we are angry at ourselves for not standing up for our truth, or for manifesting that which we create. When someone is a "pain in the neck" in our life, it can manifest as pain in the back of the neck, or pain in the front of the neck in the throat region. We allow that person to be a pain in the neck when we do not use our balanced masculine energies and set our boundaries.

Clearing one's throat frequently can be a way to move and express old fear or anger that has risen up through the chakra system to the level of the throat to be cleared out. In the same way, sneezing is often a way to express and clear out old anger or to discharge energies which are not useful at this moment in your life.

## Parathyroid

The parathyroid is located in the neck and is an organ responsible for producing the hormone called parathormone, which regulates calcium-phosphorus metabolism. These minerals are necessary for structural support in the skeleton. The association of the neck, having to do with how we express ourselves, and the mineralization necessary to feed the skeletal structure — which is an expression of masculine energy — tells us that that a problem with the parathyroid relates to how we neglect using our masculine energy to support the expression of our emotions. In other words, the suppressed expression of emotions can slow down secretion of parathormone, which can produce weakness in the skeletal structure. So the core issue here is a lack of trust or allowing emotional support from one's own masculine energies.

## Thyroid

The thyroid indicates how we use our energy source — how energy from our spiritual being is utilized in our physical bodies. A hyperthyroid condition can manifest in people who are workaholics. They stay busy so they don't have to feel their emotions. If the situation is not changed, it causes the body to burn out. Hypothyroid conditions manifest in people trying to shut down emotionally or who don't feel safe being in a physical incarnation. They are trying to put a stop to life, trying to shut down their sensitivity and receptivity, trying not to have energy to do that which they say they wish they could do in life.

# Disorders of Metabolism & Energy Usage

Attention Deficit Disorder (ADD), Chronic Fatigue, Hyperactivity, Hyperthyroidism, Hypothyroidism and Nervousness are all manifestations of not trusting oneself to be in the natural flow of one's energy. These disorders occur in people who either are addicted to mental control to avoid degrees of emotions they don't want to feel, or in people who escape into strong emotional expressions to not allow themselves the mental clarity of owning a lesson and taking responsibility for what they need to access from a particular experience. Often times, these are various degrees of shock from past-life traumas that have never been alleviated, embodied and resolved. This includes people who died in Nazi concentration camps or in village massacres, purgings or any other kind of extreme, violent death.

People who have had these experiences often create a disease or condition that makes them feel unsafe to be in a physical body. They fear having to accept whatever lesson is to be learned or resolved in this lifetime so they create a conflict to avoid having to work with the lessons.

This pattern is especially present with hyperthyroidism or hypothyroidism because these people have been severely ostracized, persecuted, tortured or killed for expressing a truth, an ideology, or an energy that was very threatening to a larger external group. So they either stay in an extreme hyper state or ultra hypo state, or see-saw between the two – anything to not be centered in the moment so as to avoid responsibility for what they are too terrified to now accept and resolve.

# Upper Extremities

## Arms & Shoulders

In our arms we store emotions and mental beliefs regarding that which we embrace or fear to embrace in our lives. The shoulders carry the perceptions of our "burdens of responsibilities."

When we feel something in our lives is too overwhelming — too heavy to bear — this belief can create experiences such as arthritis in the shoulders, stiffness or a tendency to dislocate the shoulders. Breaks, spasms and eczema on the arms can be signals from the subconscious of a fear of intimacy, a belief in worthlessness, a disgust in self-image, or a fear to embrace a new idea, choice or self-perception.

There is an enormous reservoir of body language expressed by the movements of the arms and hands. Constantly folding the arms across the stomach or chest or hugging oneself tightly can be symbolic indications of insecurity and a need to protect oneself from a perceived lack of safety in a given situation. Fears, resistance and denials about our willingness or defense against embracing our external life will manifest as any mannerisms or disorders with the upper extremity.

## Carpal Tunnel Syndrome

Carpal Tunnel Syndrome occurs due to nerve irritation and inflammation caused by the fear of reaching out to others and feeling one's feelings. This is a person who always wants to control the situation rather than trust that something wonderful can come to them. It is also a person who uses being overly busy in work and personal relationships to escape reaching inside to own and honor his or her feelings and needs. It is literally about "handling" too much externally and not enough internally.

## Chest

The chest is where we store the beliefs we *embrace* about how we expect people to judge and react to us. This mental perception manifests in the chest according to what self-judgmental belief we hold onto.

For example, asthma, hayfever, emphysema or any respiratory problem symbolize a severe rejection of self-love, coming from a mental belief system which says, "I am not worthy of love. I am not lovable." There is a tremendous expectation of rejection and abandonment derived from other lifetime experiences in which we perceived ourselves to have been rejected or abandoned because of something we judged to be inadequate or inferior within us.

### Asthma

Asthma is a condition in which there is tightness in the chest, with concurrent breathing difficulty. There is associated wheezing or coughing, often associated with allergies to pet dander, pollen or environmental toxins and pollen. This is a more severe condition than hayfever.

Asthma comes about due to a severe mental self-judgment and self-flagellation. The person holds on to thoughts that they are so unlovable and undesirable that they don't even deserve to draw breath. So they choke off their capacity to breathe.

It is important to consider repressed emotional trauma in association with asthma, especially when it occurs in children. Many children with asthma have parents who smother them with their projections of fear (commonly called worry). The child may feel insecure, doubt his/her self-worth, and thus may not enthusiastically embrace life. Instead, they tend to hide in the shadows of life, fearing they are somehow inadequate to get involved. These same tendencies can also be seen in adults.

## Breast Cancer

Refer to Degenerative Conditions on page 135.

## Emphysema

In the case of emphysema, the lung cells lose their elasticity. In the attempt to compensate, they enlarge, or stretch out of shape, and rupture.[7] Some of the damaged lung cells join together to form larger sacs. When these sacs rupture, there is the accompanying loss of small blood vessels that supply the area. This loss of the blood vessels means there will not be as much circulation of blood, the medium of the body in which all reactions take place. Not as many nutrients will be brought to the lungs, less oxygen will be picked up from the lungs, and not as many toxins will be carried off. This means toxins build up in the lungs.

Emphysema symbolizes the same issues as those in Asthma which are now more severe due to being ignored or continually denied. Issues to consider in emphysema are a

[7] Refer to information on aneurysms on page 103.

loss of elasticity, loss of flexibility (feminine energies) which results in rigidity (imbalanced masculine energies) leading to a loss of structural integrity. This means that one has not brought in sufficient amounts of feminine energies and then put too much emphasis on or strained one's masculine energies. Thus, the masculine energies have given out on them. When there is blood vessel loss, resulting in loss of nutrition, this symbolizes again that one is not utilizing the feminine energies in a self-nurturing way.

Traditional allopathic medicine may say that smoking is the cause of asthma or emphysema. We tend to see things in another light. People may smoke because they choose to repress something that wants expression and they aren't ready to allow this within themselves. For instance, if a person feels unworthy of love and doesn't want to feel this, they may choose to smoke in the attempt to push down these feelings until they are ready to work with them.

There is nothing wrong with slowing down the rate at which one works with the self. There may be a benefit in not having all issues come up from all lifetimes all at once! We are not here to judge how or when another person heals or what habits they have or don't have.

If we choose to heal on any respiratory ailments and yet we continue to smoke, it may be interesting and useful for us to see why we choose to smoke. There could be another reason than the one listed above. When we no longer need to smoke, we will naturally give it up. It is important for us to do so in our own perfect rhythm and timing, and to do it for our own sake, not for others. Don't let people "should" on you for smoking!

### Hayfever

Hayfever is a condition in which one is not able to be in the presence of freshly cut hay, spores or pollen. These are products which contain a high degree of life force. To not be in harmony with other expressions of the life force suggests that a person prefers to exclude himself or herself from third dimensional life. This person may feel more comfortable away from others.

Rather than to think of this as a form of shyness, it could actually be a fear of rejection by others. This person may believe and think, "I'm so unlovable and so undesirable that people don't want me. They will reject and abandon me." Then physical life becomes so painful, and we are so afraid of rejection that we try to reject the physical dimension. We say, "I'm allergic to nature," which translates into being "allergic" to the physical reality as a way of getting the body out of the third-dimensional Earth-plane. We don't want to be here because our self-judgment and self-criticism anticipate more rejection and abandonment from others, and that is too painful to face.

## Blood & Circulatory System

Blood is the most emotionally charged of all non-gender specific tissues. It symbolizes the nurturing, life-sustaining flow of feminine energy. As a system for channeling this nurturing feminine media to every part of our bodies, we then have the masculine structural support of the blood vessels. Thus, the circulatory system more than any other system in our bodies depends on the co-operation and balance of our feminine and masculine energies. The primary symbolic message of the circulatory system is how we use our masculine energies (intellect) to support the flow of our self-nurturing feminine energies (emotions) in reaching every part of our beings.

At the core of the circulatory system is the heart, the balance point between the mental and emotional bodies.[8] Thus, in any heart conditions, a disharmony between our masculine and feminine energies is always involved. Our intellect is not fully in love with or supportive of our emotions. We do not appropriately honor and support our own emotions, will and desires. In other words, we are not "following our hearts."

## Anemia

On a spiritual level, anemia is the body's reflection of a person's addictive belief in their own weakness and inability to handle whatever challenges or crisis they have created for their growth experience. Anemia is a call for the need to nourish oneself physically in order to get in touch with the mental and emotional nourishing required to fulfill the challenges and lessons from one's life experiences.

Oftentimes a soul who has experienced many lifetimes taking vows of extreme self-sacrifice (such as nuns, monks, Native American medicine women and Shamen) will experience anemia to teach them the severity of energy depletion these past-life vows have taken upon them. This condition is then a call and an opportunity to devote the time and energy necessary to nurture oneself physically as well as mentally, emotionally and spiritually as part of the experience of rescinding the debilitating past-life vows.

[8]Please refer to Appendix I: Heart Chakra.

## Aneurysm

Aneurysm is a condition of a weakening of the blood vessel walls, causing an enlargement of that area. The heart is usually over-burdened which causes high blood pressure, contributing to the formation of the aneurysm. This is a symbolic message of a lack of masculine support in one's life. There needs to be a more defined structure in how one chooses to experience the issues coming up in day-to-day life. This usually indicates a lack of trust or confidence in one's ability to handle the flow of events, and this is a mirror of not honoring one's capacity for strength and clarity. Also this lack of trust in one's own capacity can result in a need to control people or situations that comes not from a true spiritual attunement but rather from a suppressed insecurity. This ultimately leads to more stress and upheaval.

Aneurysms are warnings that masculine energy is being distorted into imbalanced masculine energy. Obsessively controlling people and events is not an expression of balanced masculine energy but rather the fearful imbalanced expression caused by denied self-trust. This is a great opportunity to learn to differentiate between balanced masculine energy and imbalanced masculine energy rather than seeing them as one and the same.

## Arteriosclerosis

Arteriosclerosis is a hardening of the blood vessels through plaque build-up, which represent areas of stuck and congested thoughts/ideas and emotions. In healing this condition, it is very important to have a willingness to let go and move the previously unexperienced and unexpressed emotions, especially the fear of living. The feminine energies of flexibility and going with the flow are important for one who experiences this condition. Masculine energies include those of rigidity or inflexibility, which are necessary in having a strong foundation of support. However, when one is too much in the mental body and masculine energies, and not in balance with feminine energies, the body reflects this by having very rigid arteries and veins. Remember, we all need a balance of masculine and feminine energies for health on all levels.

## Blood Pressure (High or Low)

High blood pressure usually manifests in people who have very strong emotional bodies that have been mentally suppressed for a long time. There are deeply suppressed and denied emotions screaming for ownership, expression or to be freed.

Low blood pressure manifests in people who don't feel safe to be in physical form. These people are trying to get out of the process, trying to procrastinate what's developing next so that there is not enough energy to create and manifest things. There is an unconscious attempt to try and make the self less so that they don't have to participate in life.

## Blood Transfusions

When an individual has received donated blood from another individual or individuals, there is an integration of the Akashic history of all souls involved. Aspects of the donor's soul essence integrate into the auric field of the donee.

Loss of blood is symbolic of how we "bleed" the life force from our consciousness through continual neglect or denial of our self-nurturing needs. Often there is some degree of inherent death wish in great amounts of blood loss that require transfusion to mirror a soul's attempt to relinquish responsibility for the emotional lessons that soul feels it is inadequate to resolve. Blood loss may also signal the completion of an emotional issue.

Receiving the gift of blood is one of the most powerful expressions of life. It carries with it a tremendous opportunity to renew the commitment to overcoming a fear of completing one's path that has been so terrifying as to trigger an attempt to bleed oneself of the life force. A blood transfusion is an opportunity to bring a new vibration of life to the unresolved emotional issues that need to be embraced. Donor and donee become a kind of supra-consciousness, blending their combined energies and fearful denials, creating a synergistic opportunity for a more life-affirming experience and full-blooded embracement of self-love and self-nourishment.

## Heart Attacks

Heart attacks derive from physical and mental stresses that cover up emotions not being owned and expressed. They are the result of workaholic tendencies or over-worrying to avoid the true emotional issues that are being resisted and therefore repressed in the body. The physical cause of heart attacks can come from unhealthy dietary habits. However, it is important to discover why a person chooses a particular unhealthy eating pattern. While it is important to have the most healthy diet for the cardiovascular system and body in general, the real cause of heart attacks and unhealthy eating habits is suppression of the emotions the individual does not feel safe to encounter. In this case, food is used as a drug.

## Stroke

A stroke manifests from a subconscious terror of an inability to successfully live one's life. It is an extreme attempt to escape physical life experience. There is such a sense of spiritual and/or emotional paralysis that the body partially shuts down as a result of the severe terror and need for escape projecting from the individual's mind.

Strokes can also be a desperate plea from the body to stop what we are doing, thinking, believing, fearing or expecting and be still within ourselves in order to feel and hear what our Higher Selves are communicating and connecting us to through our bodies. For many, a stroke is a wake up call to the severe imprisonment of one's fear, or over-activity to escape one's fears, and the stroke allows for an opportunity to re-access one's creative choices and be willing to experience a new attitude and relationship to one's inner self in order to resolve what the soul has chosen to complete in this lifetime.

## Varicose Veins

Varicose Veins appear as a symbol of severe resistance to the next step on one's life path. "I can't stand it" is a common thought projection associated with varicose veins. Sometimes a person feels they can't hold out any longer in their current life path, and at the same time there is also a reluctance to moving on.

The changes in direction, belief system or experience are so threatening on a subconscious level that the individual holds on to a belief that he or she is incapable, too weak or too inadequate to meet the challenge necessary to succeed in the next level of experience.

There is usually a tremendous amount of self-judgment and self-condemnation feeding this expectation of failure at the new level of life experience. This judgment and condemnation create an energetic force of contraction that causes turbulence in the vein structure in the feet and legs which hold our consciousness regarding how we move upon our paths.

In varicose veins the blood does not flow freely and there is tremendous build-up of crystallized toxins that are the manifestation of these judging and condemning thought-forms and fearful expectations. Oxygen is cut off, and the veins experience a sense of asphyxiation.

To hold on to fears of inadequacy and lack of strength denies one's masculine power, and therefore creates a sense of inability to support oneself in whatever process comes up in one's life. This denial of the masculine strength also denies the nurturing of our soul, which is then manifested as a lack of oxygen and properly fed blood cells between the heart and the lower extremities of the body.

# Immune System & Infectious Diseases

## AIDS

AIDS is a condition mirroring a tremendous fear of one's sexual history and how one relates to oneself as a sexual being. It has nothing to do with one's sexual partners or one's sexual orientation. Rather, it is the breaking down of a defense system built up over many past lives in which that defense system actually does not serve as a positive protection but rather magnetizes abusive and self-destructive experiences to further enhance the terror one holds of sexual energy.

Because there is such tremendous fearful judgment projected into the sexual experience, this has caused AIDS to intensify, accelerate and distort into the world epidemic that it is. AIDS is a human-made disease. It was created in Africa in secret germ warfare experiments carried out by the American CIA on particular monkeys in the jungle. At one point, the scientists lost control of the experimentation and the human-made virus was set loose, originally infecting nearby jungle tribes. It did not become and never truly was a homosexual disease. It was a manufactured virus to be used in warfare that spread from monkeys to black tribes and found its way to America because it was created by Americans. It was used by the Cosmos to be a mirror reflecting the hysterically rigid, puritanical and hypocritical consciousness that humans project against their sexuality.

Male homosexuality is feared primarily because of people's denial of their feminine energy, which gay men reflect equally as women. Because the Aquarian Age is the return of feminine power, it is necessary to see the reflection of this feminine power in men as well as in women. Remember, there is no such thing as male and female energies. Every soul contains an integration of masculine and feminine energies, whether they walk around in a male or female body. However, most souls choose or express an imbalanced focus on masculine or feminine energy.

Gay men reflect more strongly and directly feminine energy than most heterosexual males. This makes gay men, therefore, as threatening to feminine-denying individuals as do women. Therefore, AIDS has been used to mirror to mankind this rejection of feminine energy in humanity's sexuality. America is, outside of the Muslim culture, one of the most feminine-hating countries on the planet. The biblical excuses that Western Christian people use against homosexuality is actually a continuing distortion of phrases put into the bible by feminine-hating individuals who feared gay men as much as they feared women because of the mirrors of feminine emotions and power they did not want to feel and own within themselves.

In actuality, AIDS is a breaking down of the defense system against the ownership and honoring of one's feminine energies. The gay community has suffered tremendously from this disease because it has spent many, many years buying into the judgmental rejection by society, and because many souls who are in the gay experience in this lifetime chose that experience because they have carried tremendous fear or hatred against their feminine energy in past lives. They act this issue out in this lifetime through AIDS as an opportunity to come to a deeper understanding and honoring of their feminine energy, and as an opportunity to heal and integrate this acceptance and honoring into their Akashic experience.

## Candidiasis

Candidiasis is caused by a perpetual build-up of self-disgust over several lifetimes. All fungal and parasitic infections reflect the message of an individual passing severe self-condemning judgment that involves intense disgust in the judgment of one's past actions and assumed self-unworthiness.

Candidiasis eats away at the life force as one's self-judgments and condemnations eat away at the life force.

All fungus and parasites thrive on fear, denial, disgust, rage and all emotions related to not loving or accepting the self. While a particular diet and many alternative therapies can help balance this condition at the physical level, the ultimate healing requires strong emotional therapy and ownership. Candidiasis erupts initially in the intestines, and the intestines hold the most severe fears of emotional feeling and ownership. If the individual holds on to the self-judgment and disgust without nurturing the emotional needs, the Candidiasis can spread literally from head to toe.

Out-of-balance candida is one of the most common conditions in humans today because the emotional ownership issue is so profoundly important and is therefore the most profoundly denied and avoided. It is equally important to support this emotional nurturing and healing with a clear, positive and nurturing mental system that allows full emotional experience and does not suppress or deny with imbalanced positive thinking and affirmations.

We are not saying that all positive thinking and affirmations are bad or wrong. We are simply saying that positive thinking and affirmations are extremely easy to abuse as tools of emotional denial rather than as tools of clarity and support. The same thing can be said about the emotions. It is the delicate balance between the mental and emotional state that is the challenge in spiritual healing and expansion, just as there is a delicate balance of microorganisms in the body which can be positively supportive or negatively destructive in direct proportion to the balance or imbalance of our mental and emotional faculties.

It is important to be positive in a way that is lovingly supportive and which does not judge or deny the emotions that need to be felt and honored one hundred per cent for what they are and for what they have to teach us about our relationships to ourselves. This delicate balance is mirrored to us daily by the balance or imbalance of candida in our bodies.

## Herpes

There are three forms of herpes. Herpes Simplex is a virus which generally leaves "cold sore" types of eruptions on the lips. Genital herpes virus creates ulcerations which form into blisters in the genital region. There is also a non-genital form of herpes which can leave sores on the buttocks.

Souls who have experienced lives in which they were born into families and societies that pressed enormous guilt and shame around the physical pleasure of sex will oftentimes experience a lifetime of any of these herpes lesions. Herpes is a call from the body to let go of guilt and shame associated with sex and to allow oneself to open up to the joy and pleasure of one's sexuality and sensuality. Old judgmental belief systems and fear of one's sexual needs and power require loving forgiveness and changing in order to alleviate these physical symptoms.

## Inflammation

In general, inflammation is a tissue response to injury or trauma. The blood vessels dilate to allow extra blood flow in the body's attempt to wash away the cellular effects of the trauma. This is why there is extra heat. It comes from the extra blood flow to the area.

If blood vessels have been broken, blood will flow into surrounding tissues. When blood can't get back out of the tissues, it loses oxygen and darkens, which is the cause of bruising. Excess fluid can easily build up in this condition. White blood cells then move to the area. Fibrinogen comes in to plug up the damage in the blood vessel, producing a clot. The lymphatic system is very instrumental in cleaning up an area of injury such as this.

On an emotional level inflammation symbolizes long-suppressed anger, fear or unused energy building up and seeking an outlet of expression, but which instead of finding an outlet meets the continual force of repression. For example, neuritis is inflammation of nerve tissue, which can occur from a virus or any other factor which interferes with its proper functioning. On an emotional level, neuritis is a build-up of fear and negative expectation that is not being honestly owned and directly expressed.

Some people produce excessive amounts of histamine, reacting on a physical level to an allergy or infection. This results in very red and painfully itching inflammation. On an emotional level this is a manifestation of severe distrust of a choice that has been made or needs to be made, or it is an intense feeling of unsafety regarding something that is happening to them at the moment. Sometimes, histamine-produced inflammation can be the result of long-suppressed terror coming to the surface so it can be felt and expressed.

## Lymphatic System

Lymph node problems indicate people who *think* they are dirty, or who judge themselves as dirty, taking all the responsibility and blame. "This is something I deserve because of something I've done." Women who've been raped often create extremely congested lymph systems. Children abused by parents or who grow up in a home with discord (which could be described as a broken spirit) often have a lot of congestion in the lymphatic system. The blood is a great symbol or mirror of our emotions, however the lymphatic system is the other fluid system in the body so this can also be a mirror of our emotional nature.

## Spine, Skeleton & Joints

The whole skeletal system, especially the hips and knees, represents strength and support. When one is in denial of inner strength and self-support, then disorders with the skeletal structure mirror one's stubbornness, resistance, rigidity and inflexibility. This manifests in people who are very rigidly holding on to the belief, "No way am I willing to give up my belief system. I'm not even willing to consider another possibility. I will not surrender."

The spine connects the seven major chakras, or energy centers. The spine is part of the major "super highway" for energy flowing through the body between the etheric, astral/emotional, physical and spiritual levels.

### Arthritis

Arthritis represents one's resistance to change. This can create tremendous weakness, decalcification in bones, and can cause problems in the knees and other joints. This disorder is a call from the body to be willing to accept the strength in owning one's feeling of weakness or vulnerability, and to allow oneself to surrender to change and alternative choices in order to rebuild one's strength and inner support.

Arthritis can also be a manifestation of anger towards one's own masculine energies if we view the skeletal system as our inner strength and support and if there is inflammation around where bones join each other. We could be angry that our masculine energies have not given us adequate support. We could feel betrayed by our masculine energies. Even if these things aren't true, if it is our perception that they are, then we will have a response in an area in our bodies which represents masculine energies.

## Back

Chronic back problems originate from not being aligned with all the levels of the will – of not integrating emotional, mental and spiritual will – and not being in integrity with our own truth. What feeds patterns of denied will are unresolved emotional memories and feelings. Any suppression in the solar plexus affects the energy flow through the spine. Where there is a lack of honoring and trust in one's will to endure long enough to achieve one's goals in life, there can be major disorders erupting in the spine or heart.

Some doctors will tell you that low back problems have their origin in the abdomen, especially when there is excess body fat which pulls the lumbar vertebrae out of alignment. When we investigate reasons for more layers of body fat around the abdomen (solar plexus chakra), we can again trace this back to unresolved emotional issues. Refer to neck for related issues.

## Between the Shoulder Blades

In between the shoulder blades is a place where we vibrate the perception, "I've been stabbed in the back." This is known as the *Betrayal Point*, and it holds our memories and expectations of betrayal by others as well as our guilt about betraying others.

People who have memories from other lifetimes of being shot or stabbed in the back created that life experience out of holding onto a judgment of betraying someone or having been betrayed. The ultimate betrayal is choosing others to betray us so we don't own how we betray ourselves endlessly and mercilessly through constant lack of self-trust and self-love. Then this point in the back hurts like hell. Its message is telling us how we betray ourselves by not trusting and loving ourselves. This causes us to continue to have others act out this betrayal to us. This is a major process in the healing of the martyr pattern.

## Lower Back

The lower back, especially just above the sacrum is where we act out the, "I have no support" issue. This is especially in connection to financial worries. When we fear we have inadequate support (whether or not this is actually true), we contract the energies in this part of our body which is like cutting the energy flow or even severing the spinal cord. Energy can't move through the chakras and the body reacts with lower back weakness and pain.

This support issue is about not emotionally honoring or trusting our own inner foundation. It is a rejection of our own masculine energy, our strength, structural support and thus our foundation. When we don't trust our masculine energy, when we suppress or reject it, that causes weakness in the lower back. Especially if we see masculine and imbalanced masculine energies as the same, we will fear and reject our own masculine energy.

Another cause for lower back pain is a resistance to ask for help from others. We are convinced we must do everything ourselves because we have a lack in trust that others can do things adequately. Lower back pain is as much a call to establish a foundation by asking others for assistance as it is to trust one's own foundation of abilities.

### Osteoporosis

Osteoporosis occurs in people who are not able to allow support, who have over care-taking patterns, who allow the rest of the body to not be supported, or who give away their power and energies to everyone but themselves. Souls who tend to repeatedly incarnate as women, addictively needing to nurture others to feel purposeful and worthy, will often seesaw between lifetimes of breast cancer and osteoporosis as a manifestation of this severe rejection of self-nurturing. They need to learn to honor themselves simply because they are who they are, and not base their value and worthiness on what they do for others.

## Abdomen

We suppress our deepest denied emotions and emotional memories in the solar plexus. Our emotional memories and

Akashic records are in every cell of the body. Certain parts of the body will show us these issues. The most deeply suppressed emotional issues create an energy build up in the solar plexus.

Buddhists say the soul resides in the solar plexus, which is why they depict Buddha as fat. He was actually very thin. They portray him as fat because a full stomach symbolizes to them a full emotional and spiritual body. This is why eating disorders are most common in connection with the deepest, most severely suppressed emotional problems. We actually eat to try to push down or put a pressure against the solar plexus in order to suppress and deny the emotional issues we don't want to feel. We can also eat in an attempt to fill the void caused by suppressing the emotional memories in the stomach. When we eat to bury emotions we don't want to feel, this makes us feel empty, and then we eat to fill that emptiness. It's a vicious cycle.

The famous psychic Edgar Cayce referred to the Peyer's patches that line the inner wall of the intestines. The complete Akashic Record – the history of all our incarnate experiences – resonate in this intestinal lining and therefore affects how we digest and derive or block the nutritional energy and nutrients that the body requires from the food we provide it with. Thus, stomach and behavioral eating disorders are the most powerful and direct mirrors of our emotional condition.

## Anorexia & Bulimia

When we feel guilt about overeating, we can act this feeling out in bulimia or anorexia. These two conditions have their roots in ancient Rome. Every person, without exception, who has come to William Shaffer for an Akashic Reading in relationship to anorexia and bulimia had at least one lifetime in ancient Rome in which they gorged themselves at ritual food orgies in compensation for the emotional and spiritual emptiness experienced in that lifetime.

Rome was a repeat of Atlantean karma where feminine energy, the Goddess and the emotional body, were completely rejected. Rome, like Atlantis, was highly imbalanced in masculine energy. It was a very aggressive, controlling, dominating and over-intellectual society. There was a near-total rejection of the emotional body, which is why the Romans felt they had to control and conquer everyone.They were so out of control themselves that they projected this inner loss of control as an outwardly manifested control of other societies.

This emotional rejection lead Rome into a pattern of overeating, which was even seen by many Romans as a sign of wealth and aristocracy. Careless opulence, excessive spending, and thoughtless over-eating was an exhibition of power to them, and they often ate as much as an eight to ten-course dinner. They would serve feathers between courses so they could insert the feathers down their throats to induce vomiting and thereby keep eating. These excessive eating binges were a projection of feeling so empty and out of control because of the ultimate denial of their emotional bodies. This historical karma from the Roman empire is now resurfacing in the souls who took part in that life experience and who are now acting out and healing themselves through these present-day eating disorders.

## Excess Body Fat

This condition has a seemingly endless list of possible causes. One may manifest obesity as a punishment to the self from opulent lifetimes of obsessive over-eating such as described previously in Rome. Or, one may have starved to death in a former lifetime and one subconsciously feels safer having an extra reserve of body fat

One may be working out issues of self disgust, fear of intimacy and/or limiting possibilities for sexual partners. In learning to love the inner self, a person may choose an unattractive body. In our society today, excesive fatness is one of the most unattractive situations to create. (Though perhaps those with severe acne would disagree!)

Contrary to popular belief, the size and shape of one's physical body it is not always a direct correlation to one's diet and exercise regimen. The most consistent pattern in obesity is emotional issues one generally chooses to manifest and work through before they came into this present incarnation. Often after a passionate Emotional Clearing session, one can experience numerous trips to the toilet and can wake up 2-5 pounds lighter the next day!

## Kidneys & Skin

The kidneys and the skin hold many of our self-judgments. Self-disgust and self-resentment often manifest as eczema and rashes. The negative beliefs and resentments that we hold onto about ourselves that don't go out of the body through the kidneys come out through the skin.[9] Skin

[9] Physiologically, the skin functions as a third kidney. It is the largest organ in the body.

infections indicate a high level of toxicity in the body which the kidneys (and other organs of elimination) are unable to fully process. These simply represent the materialized projections of self-disgust and self-resentment.

The expression, "pissed off" is often used to describe anger. Often when we feel this way, without taking emotional ownership and responsibility for our life, we can manifest a kidney infection, inflammation in the kidneys, or pain in the low back over the area of the kidneys.

Kidney dysfunction and skin disorders can also tell us that we tend to hold on to things, people, places or situations that no longer serve our well-being and growth. We may contract or tighten up the energies within us when we feel out of control. This puts pressure on the kidneys, and so our bodies reflect our unwillingness to let go when the kidneys fail by holding on to fluids and toxins.

## Liver, Bladder & Gall Bladder

When we start building up rage and resentment to self-disgust, this then manifests as diseases in the liver, bladder and gall bladder. These organs take the overload when we start getting disgusted with disgust, resent the disgust, or are pissed off at getting angry.

The initial self-disgust issues manifest in the kidneys. When we react to those reactions, it congests the other organs causing inflammation, irritation, infection and tumors. The liver, bladder and gall bladder contain the most severe resentments and judgments to the original emotions suppressed in the kidneys.

## Organ Transplants

Souls who choose the experience of organ transplants do so for one or both of two reasons: (1) they are trying to remove the organ from their body to remove the emotional issue from their experience and escape the responsibility of resolving the emotional issues of the particular organ; (2) they are replacing the organ because it is so damaged that it cannot sufficiently be repaired to appropriately support them in the processing of the issue, and the new organ allows the physical support to resolve the issue in question.

When a person receives a transplanted organ they take on the emotional memories and issues inherent in the soul that originally owned the organ before the transplant. A soul will magnetize in a transplant experience an organ from an individual with emotional memories that best match the emotional and spiritual needs that are to be met and resolved. If a soul creates a transplant experience to escape the issue, it will merely be reflected back to them in the new organ and will create reactions in the body in direct proportion to their resistance or denial of that issue.

If the soul chooses to work with the issue(s) before and after the transplant, he or she will experience the support of the donor's own Akashic experiences. This will assist them in creating external experiences and/or emotional memories and dream messages that are partly derived from the donor's experience, to further stimulate the emotional processing that needs to be completed. What was compromised and threatened by the physical deterioration of the organ can then be healed.

For example, in the case of a liver transplant, the liver holds the deepest suppressed rage and resentment of past emotional experience. A person's liver may have deteriorated to such an extent that the body is endangered unless a liver replacement takes place. Such a severe denial of one's fear of meeting and feeling the rage and resentments that have been suppressed for many lifetimes will be supplemented by the rage issues vibrating in the cellular memory of the donated liver. The individual will have magnetized someone with similar issues that may feel safer to meet in the body since they are from the memories of someone else. The quality of the rage — and the experiences that trigger it — will be similar enough to stimulate the Akashic memory in the cells of the rest of the body so that there is the opportunity to feel and process the rage, even though it is being stimulated by the memories of the individual who donated the new liver.

Although heart transplants are most often caused by stress, unhealthy eating habits or congenital conditions, these are all symptoms of various degrees of denial of emotional issues, especially the resistance to self-love and self-worthiness. Receiving a heart from another individual is an opportunity to experience mirroring issues and denials from the donor. This can stimulate ownership and thawing of the emotional resistance, thereby allowing an opening up to the new heart to receive the emotional ownership and nurturing that had been long denied in both the donor and donee. It is actually possible for both the donor and the donee to absorb the learning and healing experience that the donee lives after the operation. Oftentimes an aspect of the donor's spirit integrates into the auric field of the donee so that both souls can derive a learning healing experience through the shared organ.

## Pancreas

The pancreas is another location where we stuff our "I'm not worthy of love" feelings. The pancreas maintains our blood sugar levels. Diabetes and Hypoglycemia are polarities of the same issue, which comes out of a history of "I'm not lovable." A fear of accepting the sweetness of life, the love of God, and the reality of one's lovability creates havoc in the pancreas.

There is a difference between the feeling of unlovability expressed through the pancreas versus that expressed through the throat and chest. If it's expressed through the pancreas, it is ultimately because of a basic fear of the power (and thus responsibility) that goes along with being lovable. A person who feels unlovable and unworthy of love, and who simultaneously fears the power that comes with being a lovable person, creates diseases such as Diabetes or Hypoglycemia. The inability to handle sweetness is caused by this more primordial fear of power which these people associate with being lovable and loved. This is the true reason why their bodies manifest these most disempowering diseases that greatly limit the soul's personal power.

Put another way, the body of a person with Diabetes or Hypoglycemia is severely impaired in it's ability to convert the sweetness in food into power (energy) through the process of metabolism, as a direct manifestation of the person's fear of the power that would result from taking in the sweetness of love.

Regarding the feeling of unlovability that gives rise to asthma and other diseases of the throat and chest, please look under the section on the *Chest*, and its subheadings *Asthma, Emphysema* and *Hayfever on pages 98-101.*

### Stomach Ulcers

Stomach ulcers are almost always an eruption of long, built-up denied rage and self-rage, no matter how else these emotional memories may be simultaneously projected in other behaviors. This energy becomes corrosive and acidic, which produces the ulcer. There is the concurrent issue of not being willing or able to nurture oneself because of the foods a person can not eat when they have ulcers.

## Intestines

The small intestine is largely responsible for assisting us in bringing in nourishment. The large intestine (colon) assists us in letting go of the solid portions of our diet that our bodies do not need. On the spiritual and emotional level, this system represents taking in that which we need to sustain life and then letting go of that which no longer serves a useful purpose in our life.

Thus, problems with the small intestine, such as Crohn's Disease, indicate a resistance to self-nourishment and honoring one's own needs. It can also indicate resistance to taking in symbolic messages, higher understandings or emotional signals for the purpose of releasing the false security of holding on to rigid belief systems, judgments and expectations. A deeply rooted suppressed resentment toward opportunities for change and transformation threaten the false perception of security, and this resentment to self-awakening and "cleaning house" can lead to lesions, inflammation, candidiasis and other disruptions in the intestinal tract.

A problem with the absorption of a specific nutrient can further pinpoint the exact area where emotional and mental ownership and healing needs to take place. For example, if one does not absorb calcium or phosphorus well, this is indicative of not nourishing one's masculine energies. These minerals build bones which help give the body its structural strength, and structure is an attribute of masculine energy. Now, if the mineral we have difficulty absorbing is iron, this would indicate not nourishing and supporting one's feminine energies. Iron is one of the vital building blocks for our blood, and blood is the most feminine of all of our non-gender bodily tissues. [10]

Pain, inflammation, or other problems in the colon indicate that we hold resentments, grief, or are somehow not willing to fully let go of certain things, people, places, or positions in our life.

## Appendicitis

Appendicitis is inflammation of the appendix, which is a small "tail-like" appendage at the juncture of the ileum of the small intestine and the beginning of the ascending colon. The appendix is part of the immune system. The cecum, upon which the appendix is located, is generally the most toxic portion of the bowel. Because of its design, in that it is small, it has an inherent possibility to store toxins, and ferment fecal matter. Thus, it can easily get inflamed and irritated when pathogens build up. This is termed appendicitis.

The appendix holds negative self-judgments that have built up over many lifetimes that need to be thoroughly

[10] Refer to Blood & Circulatory System on page 101 and also Parathyroid on page 95.

cleansed from one's consciousness and body. On the physical level if appendicitis is not taken care of quickly, this irritation can build up to a bursting that can poison the body to such a degree that it can cause death. This bursting is a desperate cry from the body to stop the self-judgments and to experience a "bursting free" of this self-destructive pattern on an emotional level. This clearing, besides whatever is necessary on a physical level, must include a process of emotional ownership and healing. Appendicitis is a call to balance and support oneself with positive lessons and values of one's experience as well as a commitment to no longer judge or suppress one's emotional feelings and needs.

## Bloating

When many toxins are present, excess fluids can build up as the body attempts to dilute the poison. On a spiritual and emotional level, this represents a sense of stuckness and/or a lack of movement or activity in life. One can be paralyzed with fear or terror, and the body pulls fluids into it in the attempt to dilute the toxins created by not taking full emotional ownership.

## Colitis

Colitis is inflammation of the colon. People who are ultrasensitive or who have many repressed emotions may have a portion of their colon which is very sensitive to the touch and is irritated by the least little bit of food or activity in life.

Colitis is a fear to let go even when we know something is really finished. There is a tremendous fear of what's going to come next or a lack of experience of being free of something.

Even though we may mentally want freedom, it can be emotionally terrifying because we've never experienced that freedom.

Colitis is therefore a very deep self-subversive resistance to letting go because to let go and be free is such an unknown. People with colitis can have a massive fear of change, which mirrors their lack of self-trust. When there is a lack of self-trust, there can be control issues, because if one can control situations and people, he or she feels it will be less threatening.

## Constipation

Peristalsis (movement of fecal material through the bowels) has a direct connection to a person's flow of life force in general, and specifically to the expression and flow one's sexual energy. Constipation is commonly seen in connection with suppressed sexual self-expression, where there is stagnation and lack of movement in a person's sexual energy and life force. When the sexual energy and life force become stagnant, the movement of the food material from which we absorb the nutrients that support our life force on the physical level also stagnates in our bodies.

Constipation can also occur in people who tend to escape into over-intellectualizing rather than feeling their feelings and allowing for change and transformation, letting go of that which no longer serves them. The imbalanced mental body involvement is an escape to avoid the emotional aspects of life. Constipation is a dryness that mirrors the mental dryness of over-analyzing, over-intellectualizing or being addicted to belief system, form or technique, because the emotional embodiment required for resolving the issues is too threatening.

## Diarrhea

Chronic or frequently occurring diarrhea symbolizes people who are not able to hold on to that which nurtures them. If diarrhea occurs infrequently or sporadically, it can be a mechanism whereby one lets go of toxins and disharmonious energies.

## Diverticula/Diverticulitis

Diverticula are little pouches in the colon wall. These are usually caused by differences in pressure within the colon combined with excess stagnant and toxic material in this organ. Diverticula symbolize people who hold onto physical objects, projecting purpose and meaning onto objects rather than giving value and validity to spiritual, emotional or mental issues.

People who are in the habit of being "pack rats" are an example of this pattern. This also includes people who hold onto everything they have, projecting self-value into their external objects. These people think they need something tangible as a validation of self-worth because they don't trust what they have retained in their inner experience as being enough.

Diverticulitis is inflammation of the diverticula. Inflammation symbolizes irritation, anger and rage, which results from the fermentation of values and expectations projected onto an external object when it becomes apparent that the object in question is incapable of holding and fulfilling those values and expectations.

## Hemorrhoids

Hemorrhoids are a manifestation of a deep emotional disgust towards what is being eliminated from one's Akashic experience. For example, if someone is working through sexual abuse and they come into contact with formerly repressed memories, sometimes they feel so guilty and responsible for the sexual abuse that there is very deep disgust about what they are processing and letting go of.

Especially when there has been anal rape in the current life or past lives, this can manifest as hemorrhoids as we are clearing out those experiences. There is a correlation between constipation, dehydration and hemorrhoids. Refer to the information under constipation regarding sexual dryness in life on page 126. If one has a lack of vital energy flowing through this region of the body, perhaps due to a prior sexually abusive experience, this can lead to hemorrhoids when one is so disgusted with the experience that they have difficulty in clearing it out of the body. Thus, the hemorrhoids form often from self-judgment of the experience.

## Worms & Parasites

On the physical level, these invading organisms come into the body when it is sickly and does not contain the proper pH. or intestinal flora. The bowel is always involved and unsanitary in the case of worms or parasites. In general, the entire state of the body is not strong and healthy, so the worms and parasites come in and feed off of all the diseased and decaying tissue.

Worms and parasites are an invasion into one's body and symbolize people who choose to see themselves as victims, which then opens them up to the invasion of other people's energies. It is important to recognize and own one's pattern of feeling like a victim in order to take responsibility for one's own creative choices and use the inner power to create appropriate boundaries against accepting other people's negative projections, as well as choosing to not always see oneself as a victim of what goes on around them. When we choose to continually experience ourselves as victims, we can be eaten up by other people's negativity and control patterns.

Worms and parasites can also be a reflection of a pattern of over care-taking in people. When we need to take care of ourselves and instead give all our energy to others, we allow those people to be parasites on our energy. Remember that no one makes you over care-take. This is something one generally does to gain self-esteem and a sense of purpose in life. When one focuses on others, one doesn't have any time or energy left to look at one's own issues. Then one doesn't have to feel one's own feelings of inadequacy.

All parasitic infections reflect the message of an individual passing severe self-condemning judgment that involves intense disgust over the judgment of one's past actions and assumed self-unworthiness. Thus, the challenge facing the individual is to choose another perception of him or herself, set healthy boundaries (engage balanced masculine energies) and thereby take full responsibility without guilt or judgment, and reclaim their energies for themselves.

## Reproductive Systems

The reproductive systems symbolize our feelings and thoughts about masculine and feminine energies as well as our relationship to our sexual identity. One of the biggest traps humans fall into is to perceive masculine as male and feminine as female. This misperception is the foundation of much of the struggle between the sexes and the confusion with our own sexual identities. Whether we are in male or female bodies, we are an integration of both masculine and feminine energies, even if we consciously or unconsciously choose not to tap in to the masculine or feminine energies at any given time.

We constantly confuse our physical identity and expression of sexuality with our emotional and energetic experience of our masculine and feminine energies. Whether we are in male-female, male-male, or female-female relationships, we have within us reservoirs of both masculine and feminine energies that express themselves through our physical sexual experience however we choose. Rigid religious and social belief systems and fears add to the complexity and confusion around our perception of sexual identity and the experience of our sexual energy. All of these issues manifest through our reproductive organs.

All diseases or dysfunctional conditions in the sexual organs are manifestations of our guilt, judgments, fears and negative expectations revolving around our relationship to our sexual energy and sexual identity, further intensified by the external judgments and belief systems we choose to take on from family, church and society. We do not live in a judging and punishing universe. Sexual diseases are not judgments or punishments from an external God. Rather, they are the manifestations of judgments and punishments we put on ourselves based on what belief systems, fears and denials we choose to believe in and give power to.

# Lower Extremities

## Hips

The hips symbolize the state of balance or imbalance of how we carry ourselves in the physical world and present who we are to those around us. Hip problems develop from a lack of centeredness in our spiritual and emotional integrity. When we are easily controlled by fear and negative expectation, this can weaken the balance and foundational structure of the hips. Easily fractured or broken pelvic bones indicate a progressive pattern of loss of centeredness within one's spiritual and emotional attunement.

## Legs

The legs carry the body where it needs to go in the physical world. They therefore symbolize where the soul wants to travel on its spiritual path. Where there is fearful resistance to one's spiritual path, there can be a manifestation of various problems in the legs such as chronic cramping, arthritis in the knees, varicose veins, and a history of sprains, fractures and breaks. The condition of the legs indicates the soul's willingness or resistance to the creative life it is experiencing. Nervous energy (such as "restless leg syndrome") in the legs often indicates a deep desire to "get moving" with what needs to come next in one's life. This can be great enthusiasm, a deep desire for change or fearful anxiousness that can even co-exist with one's enthusiasm and desire for change.

## Feet

The feet represent one's willingness or unwillingness to walk one's path. There are pressure points on the feet for every organ and system in body. If you are familiar with foot reflexology, you can also research the related area of the foot which has discomfort. People resistant to take the next step on the path can have numerous foot problems.Those who manifest bone spurs in the feet understand oh too well the pain of resistance in moving forward in life! When one breaks the ankle or feet bones it is time for focused reflection into one's life.

There are also times when one is clearing a lot of old or used energies out of the body and they exit the feet chakras. In this case, the entire center of the sole of the foot can be hot and can ache tremendously. In this case, it is useful to stand on Mother Earth with your bare feet and allow the energies to discharge as you feel them, own them and then consciously let them go.

Fungal infection between the toes as well as between the fingers is often indicative of a mind that over-focuses on minute details to avoid feelings and the deeper emotional issues. Fungal infections in general are representations of very old ideas, deeply embedded in one's subconscious which are coming to the surface to be healed. By combining that information with the fact that the fungus is located on the foot, one gains a deeper understanding of what the body is communicating.

The feet are one of the best areas to apply essential oils. If the recipient is willing to engage in Emotional Ownership, some people are able to clear up challenges with the feet fairly quickly.

# Degenerative Conditions

## Allergies, Chemical & Environmental Sensitivities

These are conditions which indicate tremendous toxicity on the physical as well as the emotional and possibly spiritual levels. On a physical level, the liver holds a lot of toxins and needs to be thoroughly cleansed. On the emotional level, it is imperative to be honest, and to learn to communicate that which is true.

Learn to say "no" verbally, rather than just with the body. Working with an allergic individual is very complex, since this condition may have many components to it. Most often the personality of the severely allergic person is ultra-sensitive. One may learn compassion and patience in working with this condition. The person with one of these conditions often has a fear of intimacy, a lack of self-trust, and self-esteem issues. Severe environmental allergies often indicate a soul terrified of physical existence and who wants to escape this realm of life experience.

## Autoimmune Diseases

Autoimmune Diseases are cases when the body attacks itself. The immune system somehow perceives its own body as the enemy and attempts to destroy it. Diseases in which this is a factor include Hemolytic Anemia, Hashimoto's Thyroiditis, Kidney Inflammation, Rheumatoid Arthritis, Myasthenia Gravis, Scleroderma and Lupus. In these cases, the individual is not in harmony with his or her own internal energies. Instead of working out the inner conflicts in the conscious or dream state, this individual creates having parts of the body attack other parts of the body. Autoimmune diseases manifest when a soul expresses the most virulent expressions of self-disgust or a perceived need to self-destruct in order to escape the guilt, shame and punishment it feels it is too overwhelmed to own.

## Cancer

No matter how it is manifested third-dimensionally, cancer is suppressed denied rage and extreme self-hatred that has built up for a very long time. It literally eats our bodies up in an attempt to eat us out of existence. Cancer is a manifestation of what we have judged and hated the most within ourselves. In order to fully understand what the body is communicating to us, it is important to see where the cancer is located because each area has a different message. While there are many types of cancer, the following information will get you started.

**Bone marrow cancer** reflects a rage towards physical existence . Life is defined as being so hateful, painful, awful and self-destructive that the person does not want to be in physical form.

**Brain cancer** indicates rage at a mental control that has been denying the emotional body.

**Breast cancer** is a rage towards not nurturing, caring for or supporting oneself. It is an expression of a woman's denial of self-needs. These are women who identify themselves by how much they do and give to everyone else. When we identify ourselves or completely value and validate ourselves solely by what we give to and do for others to the point of denying our own needs and identity, the result can be the eruption of cancer in the breasts. This is a cry for self-mothering and deep emotional and spiritual self-nurturing. It requires using one's own power for healing as well as the willingness to ask for support and receive healing assistance from others.

**Colon or intestinal cancer** indicates severe self-disgust and a sense of dirtiness quite often associated with past-life guilt of power abuse.

**Leukemia** manifests from feeling dirty and disgusted at oneself so severely as to poison the whole body.

**Lung cancer** is the most severe manifestation of self-rage and the most intense denial of self-love. The soul actually attempts to rob itself of the breath of life because their self-rejection is so intense.

**Sexual organ cancer** (vaginal, uterine and prostate) is the fear and hatred of sex from many lifetimes of sexual abuse. Whether the person was the abuser or abusee, cancer in the sexual organs originates in people who are terrified of sex, hating their sexual energy or their sexual identity because of their life histories.

**Skin cancer** is increasing at this time because Mother Earth has entered a heightened state of purifying and transmuting vibrational energies. This causes a vast transformation and reprogramming of the DNA and Akashic coding in the bodies of all incarnate souls. That which is left unfinished is brought to the surface of the skin. Skin cancers are manifestations of unresolved self-denials attempting to be owned and resolved so that they can literally be "burned away" in the emotional and physical transformation that is required.

People with any types of skin cancer are being warned by their bodies that particular denial issues must be addressed immediately or else they will experience the consequences of the choice to maintain the denial. The part of the body where the skin cancer appears may give clues to the particular denial issues that need to be resolved. For example: cancer on the arm can indicate something that needs to be embraced that is not being accepted or something that is being held onto that needs to be let go of. A cancer on the skin of the leg can indicate a denial of resistance towards moving on the next step of one's path that needs to be acknowledged. Cancer on the back can indicate something from the past that the soul tries to keep hidden from conscious awareness. On the face, a skin cancer could indicate a perception or judgment about ourselves that our Higher Selves request us to change.

**Stomach or duodenal cancer** indicates rage at a severely long history of lack of self-nurturing. The body is incapable of appropriately breaking down ingested food and cannot derive the proper nutrients. The guilt of self-worthlessness and inferiority are most often deeply rooted in the stomach and duodenum.

## Cysts & Tumors

A tumor is a localized area of structural derangement where the genetic DNA codes have gotten confused. There is a definite lack of oxygen and blood supply as well as an accumulation of toxic materials and cells that are somehow reproducing rapidly in a manner for which they were not designed. Often there are chemical, metallic and atomic poisons, worms and parasites. Research the tumor itself, as well as whatever part of the body is affected. A tumor in the brain has a different message to deliver than a tumor in the prostate, breast or uterus.

It is especially important to explore the emotional aspects of tumors, since they directly relate to the feminine creative energies. Creativity (feminine energies) without focus or structure (masculine energies) leads to a build-up of energies which don't go anywhere, so they can form a tumor. If we keep creating without manifesting the energies, they have no where to go. It isn't that we have too much feminine energy, it is that we don't combine the feminine creative energy with the masculine energy of action, structure and form.

Since the second chakra is the major area of creativity in the body, it is very common to have tumors in the reproductive tissues, especially if we never bring our creativity to manifestation through the fifth chakra. For example, many times a woman will feel angry, bitter or resentful at certain conditions in her life. She may be past the childbearing years and feel that there is no more use for her reproductive organs. Or, perhaps she is a young woman wanting to get pregnant who hasn't been able to. Perhaps she had a still born child, and still clings (contracts the energies) to that feeling of pressure in her uterus.

If a woman feels she's useless, she can store anger or any other negative emotion in her breasts, ovaries or uterus, which changes the frequencies in those parts of the body. Then stasis and stagnation can occur. The breasts are symbolic of nurturing and nourishing. Anger and resentment about not feeling nurtured can manifest themselves as tumors in the breasts. The woman may be an over-caretaker of others, over-nurturing others and not giving enough nurturing support to her self and her own needs. A tumor in a man's prostate can be caused by his doubting or fearing his own sexuality or virility. It can also be a collection of emotions he has been "sitting on" and not moving or expressing up through his chakras.

If you are researching a tumor in another part of the body, investigate what that part of the body does and then feel into the meaning of a congestion of those energies.

## Brain Tumors

Brain tumors are symbolic messages of the body's attempt to immediately halt a particular thinking or belief system that is detrimental to our well-being. The tumor tissue has amassed over centuries of lifetimes of holding on to particular thought patterns that are self-denying and therefore self-destructive. The tumor appears in a lifetime when the build up of this consciousness has caused the present body to feel threatened by the potential consequences of continuing the thought pattern. The body is attempting a last-ditch appeal to recognize those thoughts detrimental to our health so that a new choice in thinking and perception can be introduced to begin to clear away and transform the thinking or belief system.

## Fibromyalgia

Fibromyalgia is a condition in which there is inflammation of the fibrous connective tissues and muscles in the body, producing muscular aches and pains. There may be calcification around the connective tissue, and lack of proper circulation. Also, the muscles are in a constant state of contraction, not able to relax.

One must determine the cause of the inflammation, restore proper nervous system input and circulation, restore hydration, and take adequate minerals (the right balance of calcium and magnesium) so the muscles can relax.

When one has trouble relaxing, this indicates an excessive mental activity and imbalanced masculine energy in which one is constantly doing things and is "busy" in a manner which is not balanced by being (feminine energies) and giving to oneself. This can mirror one's over care-taking and martyr tendencies. Fibromyalgia creates a kind of armor to prevent receiving energy or information that will help the person in the healing process that they feel ashamed to recognize and own within themselves or with others.

## Physical Symptoms to Watch for upon Making Spiritual Changes

As we proceed on our spiritual pathway, engaging in Emotional Ownership, many changes will occur on the physical level. It may seem at first as though one is worse off than before! However, these changes are transient and represent the body's many inherent mechanisms for healing, balancing and "righting" itself. These changes can include fatigue, skin rashes, fever, gas, bloating, cramps, headaches, muscle spasms and immune system changes.

## Fever

Fever is an ingenious mechanism in the body. It literally burns up parasites, toxins and other pathogens. Pathogens include bacteria, virus, fungus or viroid. If we suppress the fever by taking aspirin or some similar medication, we stop the body from burning up these toxic materials. The question we must answer is, "Why is the fever present?" If the cause is infection, then clear up the infection. If there are worms or parasites, then clear out these scavengers. The level of pathogens is increased in the body when the tissue is not healthy. Many people believe that pathogens are dangerous, when actually they multiply in order to eat up the dead and diseased tissue. Does the tissue receive adequate oxygen? Is the pH. at the proper level? All of us have bacteria, virus, or fungus in the body. If our immune systems are healthy, these organisms do not harm us. Whenever the body doesn't function as it is meant to because we have improperly fed the body unhealthy foods or drugs, the germs can multiply.

Fever in the body can also indicate suppressed or denied power, enthusiasm, terror or anger that needs to be expressed more directly as the emotion it is rather than through the camouflage of fever. When the body senses dramatic change or transformation, the presence of fever can indicate a preparatory build-up of energy to allow the body what it needs to make the necessary transformation. Therefore, fever is not always an automatic indication of something wrong. It can also indicate the presence or readiness of new power or change.

## Gas

On the physical level, the most common causes of gas formation are food that has not digested properly as well as the presence of worms or parasites in the system. On an emotional level, suppressed frustrations and fears, especially directed towards everyday details, can result in the body producing excessive gas. It is often the body's cry for alleviation of worries or doubts and a need for more direct and honest emotional expression of what is troubling the individual. In some cases the expelling of gas is a way of clearing out old patterns of deep self-disgust.

## Headaches

Many souls undergo major cellular restructuring of the body as a result of quantum leaps in spiritual and emotional growth. The oftentimes dramatic transformation taking place in these processes can result in the production of headaches. The expansion of the pineal and pituitary glands (also indications of emotional and spiritual transformation) can cause intense headaches. During these times, body massage, music meditations, or soaking in a hot tub of water with essential oils (especially Lavender, Frankincense, Myrrh, and/or Cedarwood) can assist in alleviating these symptoms.

## Insomnia

The chronic lack of sleep is an indication of an individual who holds on to too much mental activity, worry, frustration and doubt. There needs to be more physical and emotional activity for balance to allow the individual to stop an addictive need to remain in the intellect. Naturally, whatever is being fretted over needs to be resolved in whatever ways possible.

Other causes of insomnia include (1) obsessive control issues which are caused from imbalanced masculine energies (2) a fear of experiencing non-physical realities – such as astral travel and dreaming – which is caused by a fear of feminine energies (3) a lack of nutrients on the physical level to make the neurotransmitters and other proper brain chemicals, (emotionally caused by a lack of nurturing the self due to an unwillingness to receive support from one's feminine energies).

As with headaches, soaking in a hot bath with essential oils (*refer to list under headaches above on this page*), body massage and music meditation can assist in alleviating insomnia. One can take supplements which supply the proper nutrients for the brain. However, one also has to do the appropriate internal work or the supplements will not be allowed to help.

## Memory Loss

Our memory is very precious to us. It gives us a reference point for the present moment. It serves us by recalling things we have learned or been exposed to before. Yet, in too many people, the memory is a constant or frequent source of frustration.

Many people panic when they experience certain degrees of memory loss associated with their spiritual growth and physical purification. In some cases, individuals simply hold on to too much mental information that needs to be cleared out as a natural part of the expansion process.

Memory loss can be a temporary experience when the body makes physical adjustments or toxic purifications in alignment to emotional and spiritual healing. It is important to not immediately panic and assume the worst, but rather allow oneself to go within and attune to the deepest feelings and voices in the body. When memory loss is a natural part of the healing and transformative process, this can be communicated intuitively through the body.

As with insomnia, depression and other brain challenges, there are supplements which may help with rebuilding on a physical level. However, one is required to do the internal work, engaging in emotional ownership, or the supplements will not be allowed to help.

## Mucus

Mucus is a thick fluid produced in the body by the mucous membranes and glands, consisting of mucin (a protein), leukocytes (white blood cells), inorganic salts, water and epithelial cells. The body requires some mucus to act as a protectant and lubricant. Too much mucus leads to congestion in the body.

It is an exceptionally common symptom to produce excessive mucus when one experiences quantum leaps in emotional or spiritual healing, as well as in physical cleansing and transformation. Especially with the opening of the third eye or the expansion of the pineal and pituitary glands, excessive mucus will for some time be produced, allowing the body to purify itself and meet the new higher frequencies of energy.

Mucus is often a symbol of long term congested denial or resistance. Therefore, when one opens up to new levels of energy, consciousness or healing, the body relinquishes its mucus in its alignment to what the soul is expanding into, spiritually and emotionally.

## Nausea

There are many reasons for nausea. On a physical level, it could be related to excess bile or a blocked bile duct, motion, pregnancy, toxins, or dietary indiscretions. On an emotional or spiritual level, it could be due to reformatting or a coding process that our bodies need to go through. Nausea can be an expression of sudden and severe terror or rage, or it can be an expression of extreme resistance or self-disgust.

Nausea can occur when one is literally "sick of" one's present life (lifestyle, marriage, job, physical location). So as with a stroke, nausea can be a wake up call. Nausea and the resulting vomiting can be a necessary immediate cleansing.

## Pain

The symptom we most commonly suppress is pain. Pain is a way the body tells us that one of its functions is not operating as it should. When toxins are in the body, they must be cleared out to stop the irritation to the tissues that are in pain.

There are many kinds of pain – physical, mental, emotional and spiritual. On the spiritual level, one value of pain is in learning to focus our energies. Pain is necessary to show us where we can make changes in any area of our lives.

Sometimes we create pain and suffering as a clue that we are focusing our life and our energies in self-destructive directions. Likewise, on the physical level, pain tells us where there is a problem in order to draw our conscious attention to that area of the body, and this physical problem is always a direct manifestation of our spiritual and emotional issues. Most importantly, pain is a signal from the body indicating resistance, and especially denied resistance, that needs immediate ownership and attention.

One must be careful not to be overly focused on trying to get rid of the pain right away. It is a signal that something needs attention. If we simply try to immediately get rid of the pain, it is like turning off a fire alarm without putting out the fire. Certainly, if the pain is at an absolutely intolerable level, then we need to alleviate the pain before we can take care of the problem it represents. The important point is, don't get rid of the pain and then do nothing else. Pain is a signal that needs our attention and not our judgmental fear, hatred or rejection. That will only create more pain.

## Remember This:

*There is no such thing in this Universe as an incurable disease. All diseases are curable. They are all caused by emotional denial, no matter how we got the disease, and they are all curable when there is a genuine willingness to own and feel all of the emotional issues that the body symbolically communicates to us that we need to own and feel. Oftentimes, the ultimate purpose of a physical disease or disorder is to supply us with an experiential opportunity to show ourselves that with full emotional ownership, we can overcome anything we have created and bring it into full healing balance.*

# Chapter 5
# The Creation of Our Lives

Most people don't like to hear this but we choose and create every aspect and every moment of our lives. We are not victims of chance, fate or external events. Everything in our lives is carefully chosen to mirror lessons, issues, attitudes, and emotions we need to own and feel in order to achieve healing and evolution.

We don't choose some things and not others. We are not victims of a random birth, nor are we victims of the genetic pool. We choose the family and country to be born into each lifetime because they provide experiences we need for growth. Some may say, "I didn't choose that abusive father," or, "I didn't choose to be born an orphan," or, "I didn't choose my varicose veins." Oh yes, yes, yes you did!

It is true that we inherit characteristics from the genetic pool we are born into. However, we also choose the genes that reflect the experience we need. Also, because we come into each incarnation with our own Akashic records of experience, abilities, lessons, and unfinished issues, these merge with the genetic coding of the family that we choose to be born into to create the physical characteristics and dynamics to set in motion the experiences we need for each lifetime. So when someone says that Joe Schmo is an alcoholic because it is in his genes, on one level that's true. And it is also true that his genetic coding is a symbolic manifestation of his Akashic record which includes all his belief systems, feelings, and denied feelings that need to be acted out.

In our accumulative experiences we live as every sex, sexual preference, race, religion and social standing in order to embody the full emotional experience of being a spiritual individual. Be very attentive to what you judge and condemn because that is a projection of what you most fear and deny. What we judge and condemn the most, we draw to us again and again.

Neither male nor female is stronger, more intelligent or more *anything* than the other. We have chosen to create societies that try to make one sex more powerful than the other. This is an illusion created from our denied projections of masculine and feminine energy which we act out in all variations until we are ready to accept the unreality of this belief. No race or religion is more evolved or has a truth better than any other. The variety in race, religion, and nationality is simply to provide as complete a life experience as possible to facilitate our spiritual healing and growth as well as to mirror the denials that we project and try to avoid. When we say that certain national, religious or racial groups will go through certain periods of time with a particular karmic issue or gift, this in no way implies any superiority or inferiority about any of these groups. It is simply the way experience is lived and learned.

## Why Our Children Kill

Why do children kill one another? We will give some explanations to this alarming phenomenon that is on the rise in our time. None of which have anything to do with an absence of Ten Commandments on classroom walls! There are medical and physical reasons that *contribute* to this phenomenon. However, the underlying reasons for it are, as always, emotional and mental.

In 1998 two particular movies were produced that most directly reflect the issues behind our murdering children.

One was a drama of such pure, channeled emotions and truth that the movie "bombed" at the box office. People were not willing to witness and experience such a clear, direct truth. The other was a film from Italy the world embraced enthusiastically as a masterpiece. Therein lie the reflected symptoms of this issue.

Toni Morrison's *Beloved* is one of the most important novels written in the 20th century. The film's release in 1998 was cosmically timed to powerfully and directly reflect a process that some of humanity now is ready to acknowledge. *Beloved* is not "just another story about slavery," nor is it "just another ghost story." A mother's love for her baby is so great that the black runaway slave, Sethe, chooses to kill her baby rather than allow her child to grow up to be a slave subjected to the cruel tortures, rape and heartlessness that Sethe herself had been subjected to. You can debate all you want about the morality of Sethe's action or whether she deprived her daughter's soul of an incarnate experience. These are not the issues we wish to illustrate here.

The spirit of Sethe's dead daughter, Beloved, returns to Earth as a young woman, still with a child's mentality. She returns because she was indeed deprived of her incarnate experience. What drives Beloved to materialize her Spirit on Earth is her deeply passionate desire to experience what would have been her incarnation as Sethe's daughter. Beloved returns to Sethe because she understands her death was an act of ultimate desperation. Beloved seeks to experience this powerful love from Sethe in order to help shift her own confusion, fear and rage towards the causes that led to her infant death.

Although Sethe strongly believes in her love-motivated choice, she nevertheless torments herself with relentless guilt as she and her family experience Beloved's presence as a terrifying haunting. Beloved needs to be present in a physical body to completely feel all the unresolved emotions to their greatest extremes. She seeks to experience and rediscover herself through unfettered joy, horror, touch, smell, taste, sexuality, fear, love and rage. And she is drawn to the powerful strength and absolute love in Sethe as a guiding foundation to help her achieve this experience of herself. But Sethe remains so totally consumed by her guilt that she cannot see what Beloved asks of her. Instead, Sethe experiences Beloved as a tormenting punishment.

There in a nutshell is the most common pattern on Earth: human souls and their self-judged relationships to their unresolved denied emotions represented by their bruised Inner Child. On and on we all go, running away from our emotions, labeling them "good" or "bad," "right" or "wrong," assigning them "proper" places in society, creating bizarre images of them in dreams as we run and run away from our emotions there too. We send our unwanted emotions into the Light, give them over to some perceived external God or guru, take drugs and keep our minds and bodies otherwise occupied so that we don't face feeling real emotions. Or if we do face our emotions and actions, it is often with severe self-criticism which only intensifies the patterns, the guilt and the suffering.

The more we keep up these patterns, the more intense the suppressed emotional energies will be as they repeatedly return to us until they can only explode as exaggerated body diseases or external dramas. Then we quickly try to remedy the symptomatic results while still not seeing what they are really all about or feeling what we need to feel in order to truly heal.

We scream, "It's too intense, and I don't want this intensity all the time!" as we escape into our pills, therapies *du jour*, or mental judgments and justifications. Don't wallow endlessly in intense emotions and dramas. It's not an "either/or" situation, although many persist in trying to make it so. We are not being chased by evil men and horrible monsters in our dreams because they want to harm us. What we run away from in our dreams are our own denied emotions that we *disguise* to look dangerous or monstrous so we can keep running. Dreams give us messages about what we don't see in physical existence. What we deny in our dreams next manifests in our physical lives and ultimately in our bodies. The more we try to deny or escape something, the more powerful we make it, and the more it comes to us and sticks to us like glue.

Many didn't want to encounter Beloved because she is also *our* denied fear, self-judgment, negative belief expectations and self-rage. However, she is also our most powerful potential joy, happiness, love and freedom. She is called Beloved for a reason. What we run away from and deny is our most beloved hope and healing truth, but we usually dare not own this. Instead we say, "I'm tired of another slave movie. It's too hard to understand and too intense. I don't want intensity. I want to be entertained." And yet, what are we so often calling entertainment? Movies which contain extreme violence in the form of killing, rape, drugs as well as the misuse of power and wealth.

We, like Sethe, must own our patterns and choices without the addictive need to rape ourselves with persistent judgment and guilt. We can take responsibility for ourselves and heal behavioral patterns without constant condemnation. We can truly learn and grow without the persistent need to punish ourselves.

How does it feel to bury dead children, to no longer know whether children are safely in school, to see one ethnic group massacre another, to lose homes and all possessions in tornadoes, floods, earthquakes, or to watch loved ones die of fifty varieties of cancer? Do "happily-ever after" movies and television shows, Super Bowl games, mall shopping, Bible-thumping, Viagra and Prozac sufficiently help?

Now we come to *Life is Beautiful*, the movie our world has so lovingly embraced. A father and his young son are taken to a concentration camp in Italy. The father convinces the child that it is all a game and that if they "win," the boy will get an army tank as the prize. Even when the child confronts the father with the truth about the people gassed in the ovens, the father maintains that this is not so, and we must play the game to win the prize. Everything will be OK, and isn't life beautiful?

Do you like this movie? Most people do. It is the perfect support of their escapist patterns. *Beloved* challenges us to face the truth. *Life is Beautiful* comforts us that we are most loving when we lie to our children and teach them to escape reality by pretending it is something else. After all, they didn't have Prozac during WWII. Just think positively and be in a different reality and all will be well. We think we are *so* loving to our children when we lie to protect them from reality!

Yes, the boy survived the war and the camp. But what has he survived into? He emerges from a death camp of inhumanity and the most heartless torture into a world of death and destruction. When the first tank of the liberating army rolls in, he thinks he has won the game and received his prize. Yes, he is reunited with his mother, and we must end this film happily so we won't show the eventual discovery that the father was executed, or that this child will never be able to function realistically in his life because his father "lovingly" trained him to face adversity by escaping into a dream world where you simply pretend reality is something else.

It can certainly be argued that the father did the best he could given the limitations of who he was and of the situation he was in. We don't dispute that. Nor do we doubt the depth of the father's love for his son. The real point is that the mass adulation of this film is not about the father's love or the son surviving. The real point is that the father's pattern of escapism is being idolized to support *our* need to escape, because we don't trust that we can face our own created reality. We want comfort that our deceit toward our children is loving and good, and this film certainly delivers that false message to us.

It will be a great day in this Universe when we choose to utilize our enormous creative gifts to engage with reality instead of trying to avoid it all the time. Again, the point isn't that the father did anything "wrong." He did the best he could in the moment, given how he chose to create himself to be. The point is, how many times do *we* choose to be like the father and use our endless belief systems, fantasies, "giving it to the light," letting God do it for us, taking drugs, or whatever to avoid the truth rather than be in it and come through it? We are afraid it will be endlessly intense, but it is the constant denial and avoidance that magnifies the intensity of it, not to mention the self-judgments that are constantly thrown in. It is not a prerequisite of emotional ownership and healing that there be pain, suffering and intensity. They are present in direct proportion to one's fearful denials, avoidance, self-persecutions and negative expectations.

Do you want to know something? Our children are sick to death of us lying all the time, thinking it is an act of love. We do not doubt the genuineness of your love for your children, nor do we doubt your intent. We simply tell you that unless we are willing to wake up and see that we're acting ceaselessly as this *Life is Beautiful* father, our best intentions will pave super highways to self-inflicted hells, and our children will be like the son at the end of the movie. Our children don't know where they are, they don't know what is reality, they don't know how to cope, they're not sure what it is they're supposed to cope with, and at the same time, they're supposed to behave in the most perfect socially-accepted way (*whatever that means*).

Our children feel unsafe because they sense that we feel unsafe. Like Beloved, they come to us to experience our strength and power, so that they may feel safe to explore, discover and express themselves. Instead, they encounter parents who either don't know how to communicate or express true feelings, or else we pontificate "family values" that do not come from the heart of innermost feeling and truth but rather are more like a regurgitating cassette tape spewing our own brainwashed beliefs, social expectations, religiously dogmatic judgments and rigid limitations.

It is not our intent to debate humanity's so-called family values. We don't espouse any particular family roles, sexual preferences, stances on abortion, politics or religions. That is for each person to individually decide. The point is, most of us rarely have a genuine view that comes from an attuned feeling of our deepest Inner Selves. Most of us just repeat what has been drilled into our heads by a fear-based cultural and religious tradition and by our fear of how others will react. We rarely show our children what we truly feel and believe, because we have no idea ourselves. We teach them that it is unsafe or rude to show directly how they feel because it makes *us* feel unsafe to see their emotions. And we were taught the same rules and limitations when we were children.

A majority of those under 30 years of age have no sense of reality or foundation of safety. These souls are like flotsam adrift upon a raging sea. You think we exaggerate? We assure you, we do not. The more unsafe and unreal our children feel, the more they reach out for extreme experiences, thinking it is the only way to find some sense of reality. Instead of us meeting their extreme behavior with our true emotional response and using it as a tool to meet our own fears and denials and thus show them this reality about ourselves, we drug our children (and ourselves) and judge and punish them because they don't live up to the expectations we place on them to support our false view of reality built on fearful denials.

Psychiatrists and social workers say that drugs and violence on TV drive children to kill. These are mere symptoms. What drives them to the drugs and violent TV shows is the sense of non-reality they pick up from their parents. This *Life is Beautiful* mentality of relying on rigid religious beliefs, family value definitions, medications, positive thinking and "giving it to the Light" only intensifies the children's sense of unreality and our fear to meet it.

How can our children ever really know if any spiritual or family values we espouse are real and helpful for them when we want to jam it down their throats like another dose of fearful belief-brainwashing, rather than mirroring it to them in the form of real emotional self-ownership and attunement? We assure you that it is far healthier, and our children will feel far safer and be more receptive, if we honestly express our fear and doubt rather than pretend that the socially accepted family values will provide all the solutions. The more extreme our children's behavior, the louder and deeper is their cry of terror and their call for help. Our children find no sense of truth or reality in our lack of honest expression of feelings, no matter what those feelings may be. Showing honest vulnerability, fear and doubt shows more courage and strength than spewing religious lessons and socially accepted family values.

There can be a mutual commitment to express any feelings so long as we express them as ours and not blame or project them upon one another. This can be done with absolutely no judgment of the emotions or labeling them "right" or "wrong," "good" or "bad." We also say to you, if our motivation is simply to get rid of "an undesirable emotion", it will stick to us all the more. The key to healing and releasing anything is not needing to get rid of it at all, but rather to accept all emotions and love ourselves for allowing ourselves to express and own them — no matter how "awful" or painful they may feel in the moment.

When we accept any emotion for what it tries to reveal to us about our own self-judgments, expectations and beliefs, the emotions serve their purpose and can heal or transform naturally. This is the key to transformation. Be as creative as possible with this process. For example, paint your impression of your feelings, compose and sing them, dance them, dialogue with them on paper in poetry or prose. You can also speak out loud to one another or to yourself in the mirror. Therapies such as psychodrama, voice dialoging and Gestalt therapy can help. Working with body massage, essential oils, acupuncture or Vibrational Remedies (Homeopathy, gem elixirs and flower remedies) are of great assistance.

If there is violence and extreme behavior in our children's music or the media, that in itself is not the cause of the killing. It is a reflection of the sense of unreality and unsafety in our children. In blind desperation, they see some sense of reality in such extreme behavior. Our children's behavior reveals this truth to us. So long as we believe *Life is Beautiful*, we can count on our children to continue their killing.

So long as parents insist on controlling their childrens self-expression out of the parent's own projected fear and denial of emotions, and so long as parents choose to give their power away to false social roles, rules, obligations and values that are not attuned, then the children will continue to kill. It's not the television that's the problem. It's not the drugs. It's not the guns. They are only *symptoms*, and dealing with the symptoms *alone* will not solve anything. What is needed for any real and lasting resolution of this problem is ultimately an inner process, in both parents and children, of the deepest emotional soul-searching and honesty. Otherwise, our children will eventually tire of killing one another and turn to killing their parents.

A lot of children in the United States today are diagnosed with ADD (Attention Deficit Disorder) or as being hyperactive. This is partly because the parameters for these disorders have broadened and become more inclusive of a larger spectrum of symptoms. Medical doctors today are more prone to diagnose their patients with ADD and hyperactivity than they were a half a century ago. Aside from this, there also is a real increase in these disorders, especially among children. On a physical level, this increase can be traced to an exponential decrease in the quality of the food that we eat and that we feed to our children. It contains less and less nutritional value and more and more residues of pesticides, herbicides, farm animal antibiotics and hormones. On top of that, a lot of our food now consists of genetically modified crops with many unknown side effects.

However, there is another underlying and more important emotional reason why we — humanity — have called the increase of these disorders into existence. We live at a time when Earth is rapidly raising her vibratory frequency. As she does, nothing is allowed to remain hidden. Everything is being brought out in the open and up to the surface to be seen and acknowledged. All emotional patterns that have been buried in our subconscious under a heavy cloak of mental judgment and suppression are now coming to the surface to move, to been seen, to be owned and healed. Our children are told this on the astral plane before they are born, and they come in to this lifetime intent on moving and shaking their emotional bodies back to full life, sometimes moving them to the extremes of what we adults label as ADD or hyperactivity.

What is the adults' response when our children desperately attempt to shake their emotional bodies back to life? We diagnose them as sick and force them to take Ritalin, a medically approved amphetamine. This drug severs the connection between the mental body and the emotional body, leaving the child stranded in its mental body with little or no connection to its emotions any more — emotions that were so desperate to move in the first place that the adults surrounding the child couldn't bear them.

Now, as those passionate emotions have a lid put on them in the form of Ritalin, they become even more desperate for expression. The children grow up into their teens on Ritalin, chemically severed from emotions that are growing more and more desperate to move, be seen, acknowledged and owned. Eventually, these children have to resort to the most extreme actions imaginable in order to break this chemically induced prison and get back in touch with their emotions. Some of the killer children of our time have been known to say things like, "I wanted to feel how it felt to kill someone." That is how desperate these children are to get back in touch with their emotions, to be able to feel *anything* again. They are desperate enough to kill for it.

Unfortunately, the more desperate our children's emotions are to move, the more terrified we adults tend to become, and the harder we try to control and suppress our children's' emotionality. Just the opposite of the response our children really need from us. This is especially true in the United States, which is extremely fearful of the emotional body. Today approximately three million children in the U.S. are being given Ritalin. A majority of our "killer children" belong to this group that we adults have forced into amphetamine addiction, while we simultaneously condemn and outlaw voluntary amphetamine usage for adults.

Why do we adults do this to our children? Because our hyperactive children reflect our own denied emotions to us to such an intense degree that we can't stand it, and *we're so desperate to stop this reflection from our children that we'll do anything, even if it means killing them emotionally*. Do you see the parallel between what we are doing to our children and what our children are doing? We try to kill them emotionally, and they go out and kill physically in an attempt to shock-start their emotional bodies back to life. It's a perfect reflection that most of humanity refuses to see, because again most of humanity does not want to face its denials. We persistently refuse to look at the reflection of our shadow side.

After all of this has been said about the plight of our children, it is important to understand that our children are not victims. On a soul level, they co-create everything in their lives together with us adults as valuable learning experiences for both them and us.

## Masculine & Feminine Energies

Let's get one thing straight from the very beginning: There is no such thing as male and female energies. Male and female refer to the "physical packaging" whereas masculine and feminine refer to energies. Whether we are born into male or female packages, we contain a combination of masculine and feminine energies.

Feminine energies refer to the pure creative power before it is manifested into form and the ability to give birth to energy. Feminine energies are present in our intuition, inspiration, creative impulse, openness, receptivity, compassion, empathy, nurturing, and all forms of artistic talents. Masculine energies refer to the ability to manifest into any form that which the feminine inspires us to create.They are what allow us to set limits and boundaries. Masculine energies are present in our clarity, courage, strength, groundedness, assertiveness, structure, focus, and in our linear, scientific and mathematical thinking and understanding.

Neither masculine nor feminine is more powerful or important than the other. One without the other is sterile and impotent. Most of us experience our lifetimes by hip-hopping back and forth between masculine and feminine energies (whether we inhabit male or female packages) rather than learning to integrate the energies into one balanced expression. Being more in touch with the masculine than the feminine can cause aggression, manipulation, domination, over-intellectualism, violent behavior and the inability to attune to our emotions, intuition or creative talents. There is a cold heartlessness that keeps love, compassion and feeling at arm's length. When we primarily operate from our feminine energy and not enough from our masculine energy, we become passive, unproductive, unable to bring birth to any ideas or forms and too easily manipulated as victimized martyrs.

The Universe does not buy into this story that males and females have certain roles that the other sex cannot or should not be involved in. These social mores are simply projections of emotional denial used to dominate and control others. This way, we don't have to face the reflection of our denials in the form of other people who live out and express that which we are trying so hard to deny in ourselves. Whether we are male or female in any given incarnation, we are supposed to utilize and integrate our masculine and feminine energies in a balanced expression. Some of us are satisfied with being in a "masculine role" at one point and then a "feminine role" at another point. Choosing to experience and live out one or the other, we can still retain the ability to be in touch with both aspects of our beings in a balanced integrated expression. The eventual goal is to be an integrated blend of masculine and feminine simultaneously, consistently, whether in a male or female body.

One sex is not meant to be dominated or controlled by the other. In any personal relationship, the point is not to be two halves coming together to make a whole. This may *sound* very romantic but it *is* perpetually destructive. The point is to be two whole beings coming together to create a greater expansion of their wholeness. This does not require role-playing. Even though it can be appropriate in sharing responsibilities that certain people do certain things at certain times, this still does not require falling into any definition or form of role-playing. We do what we choose to do in any moment because it feels right and not because of any false role, definition or obligation.

We live our incarnations as males or females to learn this truth about the equality of the sexes: The fact that no matter what the physical body is, we are to be balanced blends of masculine and feminine energies, either as male or female. Because we have not trusted this process, we have projected many of our internal fears and denials into creating false social mores and sexual roles. From this, we have then developed a dependency to be one sex or another, or we are constantly avoiding living as one sex or another out of fear of the social rules, regulations and inner emotional issues.

## Lemuria & Atlantis

Once upon a time, eons ago, the civilization of Lemuria was ruled as a matriarchy. Because the men were a little bit slow on the uptake in their spiritual awakening and development, a council of women met and discussed this situation. They came to a crucial decision that is still being resolved hundreds of thousands of years later. These women decided that the men were slower in their development because they felt intimidated by the women's power and ability to attune to feelings and creativity. From that assumption, the council of women then decided that instead of giving more time to allow men to develop, it would be better for the women to step back, relinquish their power to men and allow them to catch up in that way. The result was that the men eagerly grabbed the power, dominated the women, and have kept women suppressed ever since. This was a major karmic lesson to those souls living as the matriarchal leaders of Lemuria that compromising your integrity does not solve any situation. In making yourself less, you do not help someone else to be more. You simply become less in a passive expression and the others are less in a more active expression.

As if that weren't enough, it was at this same time that Atlantis reached its peak as a dominating powerful civilization. The Atlanteans, a masculine-dominated society, had long since lost their capacity to connect with or feel their intuition and most of their emotions. Their emotional bodies vibrated at near death. They were completely controlled by their intellectual bodies. The Atlanteans were very fearful and distrustful of the Lemurians, not understanding the Lemurians' capacity for compassionate creativity, healing and the telepathic abilities they had with animals and nature as a result of the higher vibration of their emotional bodies. And what the Atlanteans did not understand, they feared. However, fear was an emotion they could not understand or tolerate. Fear had to be destroyed. This meant destroying what they feared. So the Atlanteans decided to conquer and destroy the Lemurians.

The Lemurians telepathically received this group thought from Atlantis and knew their intention. The Lemurians, in giving all the power to men and letting the men dominate the women without maturing their emotional bodies, then reacted to the Atlanteans by saying, "We will not lower ourselves to their level and meet violence with violence." In the Lemurian denial of balanced masculine energy, they became passive martyrs.

There were ways other than violence to defend their civilization. But entrapped in their feminine-polarized passivity, they did not consider or trust any other possible choices or their spiritual/psychic abilities. As a result they became meek victims, and Atlantis marched into Lemuria, utterly destroying them. Those who were not slaughtered were taken back to Atlantis for cruel scientific experiments, or to be used as telepathic healing slaves to be studied and reproduced.

## The Battle of the Sexes

Thus began the "battle of the sexes." The Lemurians compromised their masculine energy trying to help men catch up with women rather than trusting that had they held to their power and truth, the men would have eventually caught up to them, especially when the women stopped needing to help or save the men. The Atlanteans did not want to recognize or own their need for emotional development. They became so addicted to understanding and controlling everything that the emotional body became something to be feared. Thus the imbalanced intellectual masculine energy conquered and dominated the over-emotionalized feminine energy. Neither civilization trusted itself to consider embodying the qualities of the other to achieve a harmonized integration. This resulted in distrust, destruction, control, fear and blame.

If this doesn't sound confusing enough, let's stir the pot even more. From this drama between Atlantis and Lemuria, souls began to identify feminine as female and masculine as male. On top of that, they then defined feminine as being over-emotional and masculine as being over-mental and controlling. With these mis-defined beliefs, souls then hopped between incarnations as male and female. No longer did they seek the integration between their masculine and feminine energies. They now sought either to dominate and control or to wallow in emotions, or they chose one sex to avoid the other out of a fearful expectation of one sex being a certain way.

Some male Atlanteans have later chosen to experience incarnations in female bodies in an attempt to learn that the masculine and feminine should be balanced, whether as a male or female, but they have often been unable to do so because they've been stuck in their definitions of male and female. These souls are still in denial of their feminine energies. Simultaneously, they are imbalanced in their masculine energies and have such subconscious guilt about this that they also tend to judge their masculine energies as bad because the only masculine energy they have any direct experience of is their own imbalanced masculine energy. So when these souls choose an experience in a female body in order to balance their energies, they often instead end up as either women-hating women or men-hating women, sometimes both. They project their scorn of feminine energy onto women. Simultaneously, they feel guilt and loathing their own imbalanced masculine energy which they project onto men. Since these souls' definitions do not embody a balance of energies, they experience womanhood as something disgusting, evil or imprisoning, and therefore they choose experiences to confirm those beliefs. These souls incarnate either as women getting revenge on men by trying to control them through sexual enticement, as women punishing other women who dare to believe in and own their masculine strength, or they incarnate as aggressively "feministic" women.[11] In some cases, they choose to be abused by men, thinking they need to punish themselves for their past actions. By doing this, they also try to hinder themselves from having any future contact with their inner power which they feel they have abused in their previous pseudo-empowered states.

Then we have the women-hating men who see women as the source and cause of all problems and evil. These men are terrified of their emotional bodies which they identify as female rather than feminine, and they are not about to admit or accept any feminine energies in their male bodies. This hatred and distrust of their emotional bodies is then acted out by punishing women.

Finally, there are the men-bashing men who are so rejecting and judging of their own masculine energies that they take the feminists' side in the battle of the sexes and enthusiastically profess that "men are pigs" and that women are superior to men. These men are more convinced than most women that men are the problem with the world and men are "the bad guys," while women are the loving, emotionally mature and spiritually superior gender.

Of course, neither of these extreme viewpoints are accurate. It is a well-known fact in psychology that while there are differences between the genders, the difference between two random individuals of the same gender is usually far greater. In other words, the difference between two randomly picked women is usually much greater than the difference between the average man and the average woman. Giving the worldly

[11] Ironically, aggressive "feminism" is actually an expression of imbalanced masculine energy. Imbalanced feminine energy takes the form of passiveness and victimhood.

positions of power to women instead of men would not likely make our world much different from today. Just look at the women politicians we do have today. Are they much different from the men? Politicians in general — men and women alike — tend to be quite imbalanced in their masculine energies. This is in fact the very reason why these people are terrified to *not* have power. What our world needs is not necessarily more women leaders — although that wouldn't hurt — but leaders who are more balanced in their masculine and feminine energies, regardless of their gender.

Are you dizzy enough yet? Wait! We did even more with this! Since most of us wanted to believe that masculine is male and feminine is female, this caused a tremendous crisis in women who wanted to be in touch with their masculine power and men who wanted to be in touch with their feminine sensitivity. Societies were saying men are this and women are that and they associated masculine with male and feminine with female. Almost everyone was out of touch with cosmic reality.

As a final note on the battle of the sexes, it should be said that moving anger toward one or the other of the sexes can be very beneficial to our emotional health, provided that it is done with ownership and awareness. The purpose of having physical reality be a mirror to us is manifold. One reason is so that we can look in the mirror and discover what's inside of us in a way that may be easier than direct introspection. Another reason is to give us triggers to start moving our suppressed emotions. If we are aware of mirroring and know what we're doing, blaming projection onto external reality can actually be a very helpful and useful way to initially get in touch with what's inside of us.

## Homosexuality

Sometimes people have lessons to learn from being women sexually attracted to women or men sexually attracted to men. They choose such experiences in order to recognize that whether they are male or female, they are a blending of masculine and feminine energies seeking to find the completion of the blending in the masculine and feminine energies of other men and women. The masculine/feminine polarity has *nothing* to do with male and female bodies. Masculine and feminine must blend and harmonize whether in a male or female body, and can therefore also blend between male and female as well as male to male and female to female. This becomes very terrifying to those who want to maintain the identification of masculine with male and feminine with female.

Sexual mores come out of a fearful denial of what people do not trust to own or feel. Because of this, we also do not want anyone else to mirror back the things we fear or deny. The Universe doesn't care whether we as men or women are sexually, emotionally and spiritually attracted to men, women, watermelons, or Mickey Mouse! Masculine and feminine energies must magnetize each other to an integrated balance of wholeness. This applies to everyone internally as individuals, as well as between individuals in relationships. Male or female is not the point. But humanity has created many confusing, complex, convoluted, whirlpooled rules and regulations, and then said it is all divinely directed in order to avoid not only whatever we fear about masculine and feminine energies, but also the responsibility of taking responsibility. Such complexity has kept humans fearfully hidden from their truths as they relentlessly act out this battle of the sexes.

There are many reasons for homophobia with roots in religious beliefs and social rules. They are all derived from consciously denied self-fears. Another hidden reason is when souls are in severe fearful denial of their own feminine sensitivities and vulnerabilities, and hide behind masks of imbalanced masculine control and domination. This is an attempt to avoid fear and deny the denial of fear. Some of these souls incarnate as men and some as women. These souls seek each other out as mates to support one another in the suppression of their feminine energies. These souls tend to incarnate as extreme religious fundamentalists or become involved in politics, big business or the military.

Feminine-denying men marry feminine-denying women in order to maintain their mutually imbalanced masculine control and domination. This domination and control is labeled as religious beliefs, social ethics and family values. Both the men and the women act out intolerance and hatred towards all other women and towards feminine energy in men. Energetically, a femininely-denied man mated with a femininely-denied woman is a kind of gay marriage. Thus homosexuality is a mirror to these people that they refuse to recognize. And like a bird attacking its mirror image in a glassed surface with a dark backdrop, these people attack their mirror image in the form of gay men.

Many of you at this point probably need to take a Dramamine from reading all of this, much less from creating and experiencing it all the time. There is much spiritual vertigo from this over-complexity, which covers up the simple fact that masculine and feminine energies magnetize each other, seeking a balanced integration in whatever physical packaging we are presently incarnated.

But wait! Never underestimate the human capacity to not see what's in front of its own nose and to take the clearest simplicity and muddle it into new genres of dizzying complexity. Humans are the masters of avoiding anything they don't want to see. To add spice to this boiling cauldron, there are souls who incarnate in one physical package and then decide this is the wrong package! Thus they said, "I need to be in the other package." And they come to this decision *after* their physical birth. OOPS! Now what?

## Transvestites & Transsexuals

Some people feel a need to dress as the other sex. Others go through a physical operation to change their sex. The Universe is not going to say that either of these is wrong, because they are not. We can be whatever we choose to be. But do take a look at the fact that if you have chosen to be born into a particular physical body, the issue is not to merely change that body but rather to incorporate the masculine and feminine energies into a balanced blend within whatever "package" you are in. Otherwise, you act out the emotional issues without really feeling and embodying them as you.

Again, we don't say that dressing as the opposite sex or surgically changing your body is wrong. We simply say that you may be missing the point. Whether you are a male or a female, feel and live and be as an integration of your masculine and feminine energies. If you need to dress as the opposite sex or surgically change your body, then do so. But understand that in most cases this may prolong the crisis rather than alleviate it because the basic problem is not the physical characteristics. It's about feeling and being who you are no matter what sexual package you embody.

Those of you who genuinely feel more at peace with yourselves by changing your body or wardrobe, we celebrate you in achieving that. But be very honest about whether you are achieving a true inner peace or an illusionary peace that simply covers up an inner conflict. We do not imply any right or wrong. We simply ask that you be honest with yourself. Are you acting out a role to avoid trusting and honoring yourself as an integrated blend of masculine and feminine?

We choose the physical sex of this incarnation for a reason. Whether we are male or female, we are here to experience the full spectrum of masculine and feminine emotions and energies. For some, it may truly be of benefit to change the wardrobe or the body. But for many, there are layers of "cover-up" that need to be more honestly addressed. Some are born as men but pretend to be women without knowing and feeling what womanhood really is (or vice versa) because they are too attached to the wardrobe and the physical body and aren't really living the true emotional experience of the other sex.

For example, a soul may have a karmic history of living many lifetimes as a woman who was manipulated or abused by men. This soul may then incarnate as a man to learn that not all men act the same or that masculine and imbalanced masculine energies are not the same. A deep fear of men and a rigid judgment that all men and masculine energies are the same create an enormous resistance to living in a male body. Dressing as a woman or changing the sex of the body could deny the opportunity to get in touch with real emotions and masculine/feminine issues. Instead, there can result a hardening of victimized behavior and the preconceived judgments and expectations of what is male or masculine.

We present this to you for your consideration. We are neither shocked by nor disapprove of whatever choices you make to experience yourself. But if you choose true healing and growth, then we do need to ask these tough questions and challenge you to look at them and feel them more deeply and more honestly in order to help you achieve that healing and growth.

**Women:** You don't need men to complete yourselves or to attain any strength or protection that doesn't already exist within you. It is important for you to stop identifying and valuing yourselves as caretakers for everyone but yourselves. You need to stop over-mothering, over-protecting and over-saving men. And *please*, women, do not simply fall in love with the "potential" in a man. It is very nice that you can recognize the potential in a man, but a potential is just a potential until it is put into action. Who a man is in any given moment is not the potential. See and relate to the man as he really is in the moment, and not just as his potential. You will save yourselves a lot of heartache if you let go of these addictions. When you stop needing to be needed and focus on your own truth, men will mature in the time and way that is the most appropriate and harmonious for them.

**Men:** Let go of this need for women to over-mother and over-care for you. Please learn to face your own emotional bodies and vulnerabilities, and learn to feel safe feeling unsafe in order to triumph over your fear of fear. You don't need to prove yourselves through daredevil deeds and overindulgent acts of aggression and violence to prove your fearlessness. All you end up doing is intensifying your imbalance. When you are ready to face and feel your own emotional bodies, you will experience tremendous quantum leaps in growth, and you will then help to balance and integrate the broader male/female social consciousness so that the masculine and feminine energies can integrate.

**To both men and women:** Let go of needing social, religious and political "leaders" to dictate to you what is right or wrong, good or bad. There are no such things! You are free to choose whom to relate to and how, and let others do the same. If you are threatened by same-sex attraction, let go of what others choose to experience for themselves and own that this is about *your* fear of feeling your own masculine or feminine issues.

Humans created religion to make God in their own distorted image, and the Universe refuses to comply. Our sexual identity is one form of our total spiritual expression, and we are the masters and creators of our own experiences. Religion is all too often a denial of that self-responsibility. We choose our sexual bodies and sexual experiences to integrate our own masculine and feminine energies, and to learn that they are equal and the same whether in male or female bodies.

## The Karma of Religion

Religion is one of the most aggressively self-destructive belief systems humans have invented on Earth. That's a rather sweeping statement. It is also true that there has been much genuine spiritual experience and emotional transformation within the context of religion. However, we stand by the original statement. Religion is one of the most aggressively self-destructive belief systems humans have invented on Earth.

One should not confuse spirituality with religion. Religion has little to do with spirituality. Again, we acknowledge that there has been genuine spiritual experience and transformation in religious form, but that tends to be in spite of the form rather than because of it. Religion was invented by humanity's fear. There may have been some genuine motivation to seek spiritual truth and comfort through this form. However, religion was created out of fear in order to suppress uncomfortable ideologies and emotions as well as to control mass populations.

The karma of religion is for us to eventually experience God as our purest Higher Selves and to realize that God is everything within and without. Experiencing religion can ultimately teach us that God is not just a separate entity outside of or above us. God is not a separate entity who requires worship, adoration or fear. God is not limited to a male or female body or personality. Karma does not judge, reward or punish, nor does it exert revenge or express wrath. At the same time, God is All That Is. So certainly all these things are of God too. There is nothing that is not God. Even when we create an image of God based on limitation, fear, doubt, denial, manipulation or control, still we can discover and experience God because God is All That Is.

Humans have incarnated into the various civilizations and religious forms to learn that all form mirrors the same issues. We experience different cultures, belief systems and religious forms until we are ready to accept that all is a reflection of what we are simultaneously trying to both heal and deny. We experience all the belief systems and forms and customs until we are ready to embrace our truth within us, as us, and for us, which does *not* require any confirmation through external form or ritual.

We will not say that the invention of religion is bad or wrong, but we will hold to our statement that religion has been one of the most self-destructive forms that humanity has ever yet invented. We don't say that self-destructiveness is either good or bad, right or wrong. It is simply an experience we live until we honor the highest inner truth of ourselves. Self-destructiveness is a reflected projection of self-denial. We experience and act out self-denial through many forms of self-destructiveness until we are ready to be finished with that path and lovingly embrace the truth of who we are.

So let us now say that no religion is better or worse than any other. No religion has more or less truth. No religion has a greater truth than any other, and all religions will lead us down the path of healing, hope, joy and transformations just as potentially as they will lead us down the paths of self-denial and self-destructiveness until we are ready to be free of all form and embrace our purest, highest inner truths.

Take note that we say that we experience the karma of religion until we are free of the need for external form. We are *not* saying that we shouldn't have form. Nor do we say that we will eventually be free of feelings or desires. These are misconceived religious beliefs. We say to be "free of the *need* for external form," especially as a form of validation.

There was a time on Earth when each of us had a more direct link to Mother/Father God. But as we became more embedded in third-dimensional experience, this link diminished and we experienced a sense of separation from the Universal Totality. Many of us feel a combination of rage, terror, grief and guilt at this apparent separation. However, this feeling of separation was necessary to develop the emotional body so God the Totality could evolve as a Cosmic

Being. It is necessary to eventually re-connect with this original rage, terror, grief and guilt at the initial sense of separation in order to embody the fullest healing and emotional expansion of our spiritual beings. This is our ultimate mission for self-evolution and for God Totality evolution. We did nothing wrong in experiencing the separation. Again, this was necessary in order to develop the emotional body which was the original purpose of creation, so God could continue Its evolutionary process.

As the sense of separation deepened and human souls forgot more and more from whence they came, souls experienced greater fear — and the self-denials that developed out of this fear — in order to re-discover the Light through a greater emotional experience. This was the evolutionary process God the Totality required. From this imbalance the fragmentation of masculine and feminine energies into socially assigned male and female roles emerged. As imbalanced masculine energy in males dominated imbalanced feminine energies in females, the present-day world religions emerged.

Certainly there were those who genuinely sought to use religious form to recapture answers about the meaning of life and the Universe. Certainly there were those who genuinely wished to reconnect with the original God Source. But predominantly, religious form was created by fear. Imbalanced masculine consciousness — primarily in men — dominated and controlled others to compensate for the fear and the denial of the fear that these souls refused to own within themselves.

There is hidden in the beliefs and rituals of world religions the seeds and fragments of the original Cosmic truth. Darkness is not the opposite of light, but rather the denial of it. In darkness there is always the potential of light. Although religion was created in the darkness of fear to deny fear and control others, still the experience of the form will ultimately lead us back to the Light. However, the final step will not be taken until we release our *need* for the form and instead embody and trust our inner truths.

## WICA

This is the oldest established religion, not only on Earth but throughout our known Universe. WICA first made its presence here hundreds of thousands of years ago in the ancient civilization of Lemuria.[12] It came directly to Earth from fourth dimensional Venus and entered our solar system from the Pleiades.

WICA is the most direct and powerful connection to the Cosmic Feminine Principle. In Lemurian times the initiates in WICA were trained to telepathically communicate with animals and all aspects of nature. They learned to express themselves creatively through music, voice, art and dance to interact with the forces of nature and help maintain balance on the planet. They also learned the usage of flower essences, essential oils, roots, herbs, gems and stones for physical, emotional, mental and spiritual healing for humans, animals and the planet.

WICA was the Custodian of Mother Earth and the mouthpiece for the Goddess Energy. Those in WICA were also in touch with the Masculine Principle, but they tended to use their masculine energies exclusively for taking care of

[12] Remnants of Lemuria today comprise Australia, New Zealand and Polynesia.

everyone and everything around them, forgetting to honor and utilize their masculine energy to support their feminine energy for self-nurturing.

When the masculinely imbalanced Atlantis invaded and destroyed Lemuria, the Lemurians would not defend themselves, stating that they refused to lower themselves to act like Atlanteans. They could not see a difference between masculine and imbalanced masculine energies because they did not embrace their masculine power for self-support. Hence, self-protection was seen as the same to them as aggressive conquering and destroying.

Atlanteans felt threatened by the creative healing power and telepathic communion of WICA because these abilities defied the limited barriers of Atlantean mental understanding. What the Atlanteans could not understand or control they attempted to conquer, dissect, analyze or destroy.

WICA today is still perceived as a threat to the Atlantean mindset, most prominently in Western Christian civilizations. Anything outside a fundamental belief system is perceived as satanic superstition.

To add to the cauldron, there are those who pretend to be of WICA or think they are witches that practice hexes, sacrifices and other rituals that have nothing to do with authentic WICA. Many who are stuck in a fearful Western mindset all too eagerly refuse to consider that WICA is genuine, and even less that WICA and those pretending to be so called witches are two different things. This apparent misperception and victimization projected onto WICA is part of WICA's ongoing karmic lesson: to honor the masculine power within and not give away their own power. Masculine and imbalanced masculine energies are two different things, just as WICA and pretend-to-be, hex-spouting witches are different. When the souls of WICA honor their masculine power to appropriately stand up and defend their truth and integrity, their karmic integration will be achieved. And when we all are willing to open our hearts to re-connect to the WICA within us, we can achieve a magical transformation of communion and healing between us and our beloved Mother Earth.

## Buddhism

There is a loving gentleness and openness that is most appealing to many human souls in regards to Buddhism. It reflects the truth of discovering oneself through inner stillness and meditation. It also has great wisdom in teaching one to let go of extremism in behavior, beliefs and needs. However, Buddhism vibrates an extremely heavy denial of the emotional body. Many souls abuse Buddhism's tenets in order to escape the emotional path and find nirvana through total lack of feeling and desires. This worship of nothingness as perfection is enormously self-destructive to a soul's evolution. Nothingness is not perfection. Nothingness is nothing. Souls who are most developed in the intellectual body and wish to hide there to avoid their emotional experience are most strongly drawn to the vibrations of Buddhism. Buddha taught the Middle Way. If one truly were on the Middle Way, then such a sweeping rejection of one's desires, emotions, sexuality and physical form would not be a part of that Middle Way. This is an extremism that results from the soul's fear of its emotional evolution.

Souls can benefit tremendously from Buddhism if they use it as a tool to develop self-awareness through gentle inner stillness. It can help break patterns of extremism, but not if we run to it out of a fear of our emotional bodies. When we do this, we simply exchange one extremism for another. Spiritual enlightenment does not require an extreme rejection of sexuality, desires, feelings or possessions. It simply challenges us to stop the externalized addiction to these forms. Spiritual enlightenment is the capacity to experience *feeling* ourselves one hundred per cent without needing externalized forms as addictive sources of security or validation. We can still experience and enjoy possessions, desires and sexuality as expressions of ourselves.

The karma of Buddhism is to recognize and own the fearful rejection of the emotional body, the conscious denial of this fear, and to heal the extreme behavior of being addicted to form in one life and then trying to completely reject it in the other. The Middle Way is to experience whatever we choose to experience because it leads us to feel and be ourselves one hundred per cent as we choose to be rather than using beliefs, forms or rituals as addictive sources of security or validation.

## Hinduism

Hinduism clearly illustrates the original fragmentation of the Godhead into the innumerable sparks of divine expression. It reflects God in all Its forms and expressions. However, Hinduism became lost in its own reflection of fragmentation so that the soul cannot truly feel and identify itself through all the hologramed prisms. Souls experiencing the karma of Hinduism are often extremely stuck in the root chakra. This does not necessarily apply to the sexual energy. The root chakra is also one's rooting in physical form, and the Hindus have become addicted to the karmic wheel to the point where they experience the greatest difficulty in moving onward into other incarnate experiences.

Many souls who are presently Hindu have lived Hindu incarnations for 75 per cent or more of their incarnations over the past 3000 years. The Hindus celebrate how wonderful it is when a child can remember that in his previous life he was the son of so-and-so in the next village 50 miles away. What they do not recognize is that many of them simply reincarnate from one village to the next, life after life, worshipping the karmic wheel rather than moving through it. Yes, it's nice and can be of help to recall past-life memories, but it is not a sign of spiritual evolution to do so. Most Hindus are addicted to the phenomenon of reincarnation rather than getting on with it. And although a human soul can choose to reincarnate as an animal, 99% of the time they do not because that is not a step forward. A cow need not be sacred because it could be our old grandfather. A cow is sacred because it is a cow!

It is far better to focus on what we feel in each moment of life experiences and what those feelings reflect to us about our perception and conscious choice of ourselves rather than glamorize our ability to recognize past lives. Hindus have created such a vast circus of Gods and Goddesses that they have lost themselves in the maze of characters. Again, this reflects the true fragmentation of the Godhead in all Its forms. But the Hindus do not internalize their belief structure enough, and so they go round and round the karmic porridge, returning to their Hindu belief systems and culture again and again without moving forward. Souls in the Hindu vibration need to move into their inner feelings and honor the equal divinity of their masculine and feminine energies, and spend less time cruising the pantheon of Gods and Goddesses or their past-life journeys in the surrounding villages.

## Judaism

Judaism came to Earth from a far distant star system to anchor the third eye energy in Earth. The Jews were bringers of cosmic wisdom and law, and they chose to act out the karma as the conscience of humanity. Thus they lived archetypal experiences that became the foundation for later civilizations and religions and set the stage for the journey to one's soul conscience. However, over the centuries they have become so addicted to the word and the law that sometimes they can't see the temple for the pillars. Although there is tremendous creative passion in Judaism, quite often an addiction to the law consciousness has overshadowed this energy, and it has then taken severe crises to bring the creative passion back into an equal expression.

There are those who like to stereotype the Jews as being "the ones with the guilt"! However, it is not the Jews who came up with the belief system that humans are born in sin. This was a Christian concept, and to be born in sin is about as guilt-ridden a trip as you can lay on anyone! Guilt is something all religions karmically share together. Then there are those who say the Jews are "the great martyrs," even though it is the Christians who worship the martyrs and it is the Muslims who celebrate dying as martyrs fighting against the infidels. Martyrdom is also shared by all the religions. But because the Jews chose to accept the karmic role as the conscience of humanity, they do act out and reflect what appears to be an extraordinary amount of suffering because they reflect the fearfully-denying choices of all of humankind.

Many souls choose to experience lifetimes as Jews when they have been expressing intolerance and persecution towards other religions, races or cultures. Because so much has been projected and blamed upon the Jews, it became a vibration into which many souls tried to punish themselves by experiencing the punishing intolerance of other groups. The karma of the Jews is to no longer need to be this suffering mirror for the other religious groups, but to simply take responsibility for themselves and allow the other groups to take responsibility for their own.

Many souls accuse the Jews of extreme arrogance because they are called "the chosen people," and because of their willingness to argue God to Its face. Most other religions are appalled and terrified at this ability to question God. And yet we say that this is one of the greatest gifts Judaism has to teach the world. God is not just an external being who wants to be a puppet-master pulling our strings. If we do something simply because God demands or commands it, it has no point. Many consider it sacrilegious that Jews don't believe in a middleman and are willing to dialogue, debate and outright argue with God. To think that anything is sacrilegious is one of the great hoaxes invented by humanity. God the Totality wants us to dialogue and debate and argue as part of the process of discovering and creating our own truths.

When the Bible refers to the Jews as the chosen people, this is not meant to imply an elitism or superiority. It simply refers to a cosmically historical fact that the Godhead chose a group consciousness from a different star system to come to Earth as a catalyst of humanity's conscience and to bring a new order of law and understanding to the planet. But so much fearful resistance and denial has been projected upon the Jews that their karma has been distorted into acting out scapegoatism and martyrdom, especially by souls who are born into this vibration to punish themselves for past-life intolerance. The original vibration of Judaism became distorted by this phenomenon.

## Christianity

The original karmic intent of Christianity was to bring a heart chakra balance to Judaism which had become trapped in the mentality of the Jewish law. But imbalanced masculine energy destroyed Christianity from its very beginning, and instead it became one of the most heartlessly destructive experiences on Earth. Christianity's karma is to bring the heart message of grace through self-forgiveness and to bring out the love and joy inherent in one's own heart. This became distorted into grace through an external savior, with love and joy being rammed down peoples' throats through intolerant persecution and violence.

No religious form has been more persistently violent and destructive — a religion originally manifesting from the heart chakra. But therein lies the ultimate karma of Christianity. When we do not feel and honor the truths of our own hearts, we become addicted to external suffering, martyrdom and a savior to be worshiped for suffering for us.

Yeshua's[13] crucifixion was an archetypal enactment of a soul's ongoing self-crucifixion through earthly incarnations until it is ready to own and heal its persistent addiction to self-denial and worthlessness. Yeshua did not suffer and die for us. He did not take anybody else's karma upon himself. His crucifixion merely mirrored to the rest of us how we repeatedly sacrifice and give up our own power and crucify ourselves in the misbelief that such things are acts of love. Believe us when we say that God would never consider it an act of love to choose a soul to suffer and die for anyone. We hang on our own crosses of self-denial until we accept that every moment we live is self-chosen and self-created in order to teach us that we are one hundred per cent our own masters, creators and saviors.

This is the ultimate heart message that Christianity was meant to give, which got buried by the imbalanced masculine energy of the people who established the Christian church. Their fear of their feminine energy, their fear of women, their need to be free of Rome, and their need to control everyone around them created a church of heartless rules and intolerance that was the antithesis of heart's intended message.

Nevertheless, light still lives in the darkness. Through experiencing the karma of Christianity, souls learn to meet the depth of their self-denial. This will lead to the understanding that separation from God was an illusion necessary to develop the emotional experience of self, which will give birth to the true grace of one's own heart, re-embracing the total light of God within.

---

13 There was never anyone called Jesus. Jesus is a Greek name. They spoke Aramaic in Israel 2,000 years ago, and his name was Yeshua Ben Yosef.

## Islam

Islam was created out of the world's rage towards the extremely destructive intolerance of the Christian church. Islam burns with self-righteous rage against religious intolerance. The original intent of Islam was to be a purifying phoenix flame, catalyzing souls into waking up from their stupor of being controlled and victimized by the church. For a brief time (8th-15th centuries), the Moorish occupation of southern Spain was the greatest illumination of the Islamic karma. The Moors began to bring Europe out of the dark ages when they shared the light of their wisdom and tolerance. When the Christian church succeeded in throwing them out of southern Spain in 1492 and replaced them with the ultimate cruelty of the Inquisition, the rageful hurt of the Moors was so intense that it distorted the flame of Islam into an extremely revengeful intolerance that has been reacting to Christianity ever since. They were so hurt and disgusted by Christianity's reaction to their tolerant wisdom that they themselves became what they hated the most in Christianity.

Today Islam continues to be primarily this pained, grieving, revengeful reaction to Christianity. They have mirrored and carried to an even greater extreme a tormenting rejection of feminine energy, especially as they see it symbolized in women. They have become a religion of reaction rather than inner being. There is much heart forgiveness that needs to take place in Islam if it is to have any chance of returning to its greatest glory as expressed through the Moors in southern Spain. If they continue to hold on to their revengeful hatred, the flame will consume them and their countries until there is nothing left but an Armageddon of ash.

## Scientology

Is Scientology the evil bogeyman stealing millions from its followers, practicing horrific brainwashing, threatening those who leave the organization, and projecting curses on those who speak out against it? Certainly we have heard from hundreds who say so, and we can only say that it is up to each to attune within as to the truth of these stories about Scientology. Definitely we have witnessed many in this organization who have achieved enormous success and wealth and attribute it to the philosophy of this organization. There is tremendous mystery and innuendo, accusations and success surrounding Scientology.

Karmically speaking, we can only say that there is something insidious within the organization that will eventually be pulled into the total light of day. Souls drawn into this experience magnetize to themselves the karmic lesson to not focus on the kind of external achievement gained through practicing the tenets of Scientology. Their lesson is to open their physical and inner eyes to all that goes on within the organization and not be blind to anything not truly of the highest good. There is something to be learned here about feeling and being who you are within the process rather than focusing on desired end results. Turning a blind eye to possible distortions and abuses within an organization because it is simply not happening to you is one of the main karmic lessons Nazi Germany had to mirror to humanity. We do not equate Scientology with Nazi Germany, but we reflect to the followers of this organization that the behavior of the Germans (and most of the world at that time, for that matter) has much to teach and warn them as a valuable mirror of karmic experience.

## Science of Mind, Unity, Eckankar, Church of Religious Science

Science of Mind, Unity, Eckankar and the Church of Religious Science provide much positive support. Although there is much inherent spiritual truth in these groups, the primary karmic lesson here is that they are over-focused on positive thinking as a denial of emotional ownership and expression. We don't deny the spiritual truths they express, but knowledge of spiritual truth is not enough. One does not evolve merely by knowing, understanding or accepting anything. Spiritual growth derives primarily from emotional feeling and from *being* the truth of who we are.

These spiritual groups generally aim for a quick fix and ascension, which will not be achieved by belonging to a group or knowing anything. Ascension is the natural result of the full embodiment of being. The karma of the souls in these groups is to not try to find the fastest way to anything, but rather to take full self-responsibility and ownership and be grounded in the reality of their personal experience, rather than flying away into either airy-fairy New Age escapism or into dogmatic belief systems.

## Atheism & Agnosticism

We will also say to those who are atheists and agnostics that you are sometimes the most profound spiritual pioneers because you are willing to perceive and experience beyond the limitations of religious form. We will also say that many atheists and agnostics are not being completely honest when they say they do not believe in God. What is more correct is that they do not believe in any religious definition of God, and we highly celebrate them for this. Do not confuse a lack of belief in a religiously defined God with a lack of belief in God.

Though if you still do not believe in God, don't fret about it. God does not require your belief or adoration. God *is* regardless, and God is all and everything, however you define that. Totality is your ultimate responsibility as a spiritual being. Even if you choose to believe that the Universe is completely accidental and random, this does not prevent the experience and expansion of love in your heart. So long as you are open to love, honor yourself as a unique spiritual being, and are willing to at least respect your fellow human beings in whatever beliefs or forms they have, this will lead you to the grace of your inner heart. Grace does not require belief. Love does not require belief. Love requires only feeling and being. Let this be the comfort and the guiding light to your highest spiritual evolution.

Everyone has the responsibility to choose how to experience and define spirituality. Choose and experience religious form or not. There are kernels of light and truth in all religions. But they were established with a lot of fear and an imbalanced masculine need to dominate and control through one form or another. Those who have achieved genuine spiritual transformations through religious form often do so because of something inherent within themselves far beyond the religious form. Certainly aspects within the religious form can act as catalysts, comfort or guideposts, but the ultimate karma is to pass through all religious form and see that they are all intrinsically the same and equally limited in their fear-based foundations. Hold to a religious belief, whatever it may be, so long as you feel the need to. Hopefully, you can discover the grace of God in your own heart, which is not limited or determined by any religious belief or form. That is the ultimate karma of religion.

## The Karma of Race & Nationality

There are multitudes of races and nationalities on Earth. Part of the reason is because we were seeded by various extra-terrestrial species, although ultimately we all share a root origin of One Consciousness. The other reason for the vast variety of races and nationalities is to make it possible to experience all facets and variations on the karmic themes to ultimately teach us that everything is one and the same.

We will state clearly at this point that no race or nationality is superior to another. No race or nationality has a greater truth or mission than another. No race or nationality is of any higher quality or vibration than any other. You incarnate through the various races and nationalities to experience your self in all the facets possible in order to evolve into the highest vibration that you can experience in this dimension. Whereas it is true that there are different variations on the karmic themes in the different races and nationalities, one is not better than any other. They are simply different experiences to give us a well-rounded achievement and assimilation of your self.

***Ultimately, the karma of all races is that there is only one race: the human race.***

*No matter what color the skin, no matter what star system anyone came from, no matter what cultural, political or religious history, there is only one race. Our "karmas of the races" is an illusion of separation derived from lack of self-love, lack of trust in our internal spiritual power and by an externalization of God from our own inner ownership.*

*We create and act out the illusion of multiple-race karmas until we are ready to choose to not be threatened by a sense of unity. Many believe Oneness denies individual identity. This is not true. Separation supports a sense of identity based on fear. Ultimately we must trust to accept that we are individuals and one simultaneously without separation.*

## The Red Race

The red race first emerged on Earth in the Atlantean culture. They came to Earth to be the custodians of the planet. Their mass consciousness vibrated a special telepathic and emotional bonding with Mother Earth that enabled them to care-take the planet as they proceeded with their own karmic experience. As Atlantis progressed and this group consciousness became more grounded in third-dimensional energies, they began to lose conscious connection with their spiritual origin and became more attached to creating, owning and mastering physical things. After the destruction of Atlantis, some of the souls had accumulated enough karmic experience to choose to return to the Earth connection and custodianship. Others maintained their addiction to production, ownership and mastership of the physical plane and continued to become more caught up in that experience.

Those of the red race who learned from their Atlantean experience and returned to a deeper commitment and custodianship of the Earth then returned again and again to those cultures we today know as the Native American cultures of both North and South America, including the Inuit (Eskimos). Thousands of years ago, the red race also inhabited large portions of the Eurasian landmass. One of the characteristics of the red race is a low birth rate, and as the white, yellow and brown races multiplied beyond their bounds, the red race nearly disappeared from the Old World. Some nationalities of the red race that still survive in Eurasia include the Sami (Lapps) of Scandinavia and many of the numerous indigenous tribes of Siberia and the Altai region of Russia. The red race is the race that is most varied and indistinct in its physical appearance. Fragments of the Earth custodians of the red race are also scattered throughout more temperate and tropical regions of the Old World as "indigenous tribes," such as the Vedda of Sri Lanka and the Ainu of northern Japan. The Mongols are a hybrid between the red and yellow races. In appearance they resemble the yellow race, but culturally and spiritually they are closer to the red race.

Although there has been profound dedication and heart connection to Mother Earth among the red race, there has continued to be a lack of self-identity and commitment with the same dedication and heart connection to themselves as spiritual beings. They created belief systems and rituals to celebrate and bless the Earth, but to the point of emotional denial of their own individual karmic process. Thus the red race ultimately magnetized to itself the "victimization" by the white race, not as a judgment or punishment of this denial (although it certainly felt that way in their experience), but as a mirror of their severe denial of their own individual self-commitment.

Cosmos does not question or invalidate their heart-felt commitment and integrity toward Mother Earth, but without relating in the same manner toward themselves, their energies ultimately distort and become self-destructive. The red race today needs to heal its perception of victimization, take responsibility for the mirroring the white race acted out for them, and re-dedicate themselves to a path of emotional ownership and self-healing that is of an equal vibration with their commitment to Mother Earth.

Mother Earth is not pleased with the growing number of casinos on the lands of the red race. This is not because She would deny them the financial resources, but because there is tremendous impure motivation behind this creative choice. There is much revenge against the white race in this, and the denial of this motivation of revenge blocks them from the ownership and healing of their feeling of victimization and their own self-denials. Until this is appropriately resolved, the consciousness that vibrates from these casinos builds up to a maelstrom of crisis and suffering that they will have to endure. Again, this is not as a judgment or punishment, but as the consequential reflection of their continuing denial-perception of victimization and impure motivations.

## The Brown Race

The brown race encompasses the India Indians, the Nepalese and other Himalayan people, most Indonesian ethnic groups, Polynesians, Melanesians, Aborigines, Maori and others. The Tibetans have their roots in the brown, red and yellow races, with distinct characteristics of all three groups.

The brown race appeared on Earth through the civilization of Lemuria. Like the red race, they too were committed to Earth custodianship and were also the manifestors of various healing arts through the creative expressions of music, dance and art. There is a tremendous dedication to the Goddess energy that has been maintained throughout their physical history on this planet. But they lacked an equal dedication to, and trust of, their masculine energy, which resulted in their ultimate destruction by the Atlanteans.

Even into the time when this book is written, the brown race still acts out an extreme rejection of their masculine energy that causes them to be dominated and exploited by the imbalanced masculine energies of other races and nationalities, especially by the Americans, the British and the Muslim culture. They carry within themselves the tremendous compassionate power potential of the Goddess. There is much the brown race has to re-teach the rest of the planet about experiencing and expressing the feminine capacity to nurture and heal through creative expression. But they must learn to emotionally trust their balanced masculine energy and see that it is not the same thing as imbalanced masculine energy. When they are ready to stop being manipulated by the mentally and capitalistically dominated Western culture, they can then take their rightful place as equal co-creators on this planet.

## The Black Race

The original inhabitants of sub-Saharan Africa and their descendants in the New World constitute the black race.

Most of the tribes of Ethiopia, Eritrea, Sudan and Somalia are a mixture between the black and the white races. The black race came to Earth from the Sirian star system[14]as the most highly developed and full-bodied emotional expression of Spiritual Being. Especially in the areas of music, art, dance, voice and all aspects of creativity, this group has excelled in the levels of joy, compassion, oneness with nature, spiritual wisdom and healing energies manifested in this dimension of reality.

It is precisely because of these emotionally and spiritually dynamic qualities that this karmic group has repeatedly provoked, irritated and threatened other cosmic civilizations that are in deep emotional denial. Through imbalanced masculine domination, these other groups have pursued, attacked, persecuted, and often massacred the soul group that exists on Earth as the black race. This soul group has been continually attacked, enslaved and killed for existing as a powerful vibration of emotional embodiment and Heart Light by many other soul groups who felt threatened by the black race's strong vibration. Over the eons the soul consciousness of the black race has taken on deep-rooted emotional scars of insecurity, inferiority, paranoia, victimization and desire for revenge.

This soul group is learning — and hopefully teaching others — to never deny or compromise itself by being less for the sake of accommodating the fearful denials and judgmental projections of others. At the same time, there is the often painful journey towards owning their own patterns of

---

[14] When a race's extraterrestrial origin is mentioned, it primarily refers to the origin of the group consciousness rather than to a physical origin, even though there is also some actual genetic E.T. involvment in the human gene pool.

denying their self-value and self-love, and how this self-rejection has magnetized the constant attacks and suppression of them through countless planetary experiences.

As with the red race group experience, the Cosmos celebrates the magnificent emotional embodiment, creativity, spiritual wisdom and loving capacity of these Beings. However, their love and creative expression has predominantly been given *out* to an external perception of God to the point of denying these abilities and powers for their individual inner selves. Along with the red race, their karma has been to love *themselves* as much as they express love to all that is *around* them. It also involves honoring their talents as *aspects* of themselves that stem *from* themselves rather than as something that merely comes *through* them *for the sole benefit of someone or something outside of themselves.*

Being able to let go of the continued magnetization of their victimization — and the resulting martyrdom — is dependent upon this. To do so requires the black race to come to terms with their addiction to victimization. It is important to find a willingness to take responsibility and heal this without further self-judgment and punishment, and without the need for projecting continual blame on the race(s) who mirrored their lack of self-love. There is absolutely nothing inferior or less about the group consciousness of the black race. It is simply a matter of allowing themselves the time, space and experience to go as deeply within themselves as possible to liberate their untapped potential and allow it to be expressed to the surface of their consciousness and bodies in an equality with the other races.

Through all the relentless and heartless tortures and inhumane cruelties thrust upon the blacks as slaves, they were never truly slaves in their souls. An absolute connection and emotional/spiritual embodiment with The One maintained a dignity, strength and courage that the slave owners could not shatter. This was extremely threatening to the white race who was often very heartless, mentally dominated and disconnected from nature. There was only one solution to breaking the power of the black race's spirit — impose upon them the religion of their white "owners". Once the blacks embraced Christianity, they were truly enslaved in the rigid, intolerant, emotionally and feminine-denying belief system that told them, "You are *supposed* to suffer here. Good people suffer. Your reward is somewhere other than here. Be meek and humble. Do not question, simply accept your fate." *That was the true enslavement of the black race.*

On the other hand, Cosmos used the intolerant domination of the white Christian consciousness to bring the blacks into the vibratory field of Christianity for a higher purpose — to infuse the Christian energy field with full-bodied emotional power, compassion and healing love. It has been extremely painful for the black race to bring this gift of emotional being to the Christian vibration. However, it is a vital opportunity for all souls concerned to learn how victim and victimizer mirror two sides of the same coin. It is equally important to see how addiction to blame reflects a lack of self-value, self-trust and self-love. Through the continuing life experience all souls may learn, evolve and heal.

There is a particularly interesting pattern expressing itself on Earth at this time in regards to the black race and most specifically with the black women of the United States. Souls who have chosen to incarnate as black women in the United States over the past 100 years have chosen a karmic mission of being powerful transmitters and manifestors of the highest heart chakra energies. This pattern is predominant in the United States because this country is at present the most powerful and influential culture on the planet, and at the same time one of the most heartless and fearful towards feminine energy on Earth.

Black women in America have taken on a special mission of striving to greater heights in wisdom, compassion, healing and heart power through writing, music, theater and the nurturing of their own families as well as white families. Black women anchored healing light and love for their race in their service of tending white homes. It is because of these black *women* that Martin Luther King was able to carry out his mission as he chose to, as well as all the accomplishments in the civil rights movement. These souls living as American black women have grounded more heart energy into the United States than any other race or national group. America has not yet awakened to the reality of these powerful women and what it owes them for what they experience and manifest upon Earth.

At this present time there are specifically three Afro-American women who anchor into the human consciousness the most powerful heart energies and opportunities for spiritual awakenings. Maya Angelou is a manifestation of Divine heart chakra. Her poetry and other writings vibrate the highest level of spiritual wisdom and compassionate healing experienced on the Earth plane.

Toni Morrison's books are among the most important books of the 20th century. Her three books — *The Song of Solomon, Beloved and Paradise* — offer a complete experiential process of a soul's journey through self-discovery, inner-integrity, emotional ownership, and the most holistic spiritual healing. *Beloved* is one of the most important novels written during the 20th century, as it deals most directly with our need to journey inwards to meet, embrace, own and heal the wounded inner child, battered and abused by our guilt, judgments and rigid belief systems.

Iyanla Vanzant[15] is one of the most profound spiritual teacher/healers on the planet. Her books and lectures offer the deepest and most compassionate process of self-discovery forgiveness, and healing. These three women form a trinity of spiritual power anchored into the Earth vibration and human consciousness, and the more people allow themselves to be exposed to these women's truths and energies, the greater the potential for spiritual awakening and expansion.

These three women, along with the mass consciousness of Divine compassion that particularly manifests so strongly through the souls of Afro-American women, offer a powerful dynamic opportunity for human healing and development and also act as an important counter-balance against the aggressively denied rage and blame of Louis Farrakhan and his Nazi-like Nation of Islam.

We also choose to add a special comment about Oprah Winfrey. Because of her enormous popularity, Oprah is one of the most influential individuals of our time. Through her screen acting and work on television, she serves as a conductor of heart-balanced spiritual wisdom to the masses of our Western society on a scale that has never before been seen. We acknowledge her wisdom, her own personal inner growth as a result of her work which she willingly shares with the world, and her commitment to healing the emotional body.

In contrast to this, there is the collectively denied blaming rage of the black race that Louis Farrakhan and Nation

[15] Most famous through her many appearances on Oprah Winfrey's television shows.

of Islam are holding, which can only be healed when the individuals of the black race own and heal this blaming rage within themselves. Denying that we have any blaming rage may *seem* more loving — and the black race is by nature very warm-hearted and loving — but the only truly loving thing to do is to bring all denied aspects of us back into ourselves and heal them within.

When we deny our fear-based emotions, they go outside of us and wreak havoc in a state of denial. Our denied emotions can actually leave our energy fields and attach themselves to others who will accept them. Thus, much of the collectively denied blaming rage of the black race has left the individuals who denied having it and is now clustered around Farrakhan and his followers, supporting and empowering them in their already acknowledged blaming rage toward the other races and religions.

Farrakhan and his followers do not, however, have the power to heal this blaming rage because most of it was never theirs to begin with. Any denied emotion can only be healed through being taken back and owned by the individual in whom it originated. When the individuals who denied this blaming rage take it back in order to acknowledge, own and heal it, then it will not have to be acted out as violence and aggression in a state of denial.

Cosmos certainly understands the intensely painful rage of the group consciousness of the black race. However, all souls must learn that they are not the victims of one another but rather responsible choosers and creators of their own destinies, and that all of humanity mirrors this denied truth. All souls must take responsibility for their creative choices without any further self-imposed guilt and need for judgment and punishment. The black race as a group consciousness has chosen to act out this mirror to all of humanity as they heal this wound within themselves and take responsibility for their own power and destiny without the need for externalized blame and aggressive attack.

Seek the books and televised interviews and lectures of Maya Angelou, Toni Morrison and Iyanla Vanzant, as well as the work of Oprah Winfrey, and embrace the compassionate power, grace, strength and loving immensity that these women as Goddess manifestations mirror to all of humanity.

## The Yellow Race

The yellow race is primarily made up of the people of China, Indochina, Japan and Korea. People of the yellow race, especially of the Chinese nationality, also live as distinct sub-cultures in most other countries of the world.

The yellow race comes from planetary systems outside this galaxy and came to Earth with great cosmic wisdom and power. In their manifestation of the Chinese culture, they were the only other advanced civilization on Earth contemporary to Atlantis, and they are the only civilization on Earth that has continued uninterrupted since Atlantean times. The yellow race has always been highly evolved intellectually and great masters of artistic expression, and their karma has always been to develop their individuality rather than depend solely on group consciousness. In other star systems, when the yellow race has manifested on planets not of humanoid form, they have appeared in what is closest to the biological forms of insects. One can still see in their oriental cultures great similarities to insect-like colonies.

This is not meant to be any kind of a negative judgmental statement. There is no implication of wrongdoing or inferiority in this. It is simply that the yellow race in its cosmic history has put more importance on group consciousness to a severe degree of denying individuality. In this the insects of Earth mirror them. The orient reflects the ant colony or beehive in many ways. Through their interfacing with the other races and cultures on Earth, they are here to learn to maintain their high quality of intellect and culture, but not to the degree of denying individualism. They are here to learn to celebrate the uniqueness of the individual and to experience that individuality does not automatically compromise the greater good of the whole. There is much the rest of the world can learn from the yellow race about greater cooperation and integration in communal experience.

Much of the conflict between the East and the West has been the West's over-glorification of the individual to the point that it damages group dynamics versus the East's over-glorification of the communal consciousness to the point that it severely denies individuality. Just as we have the Atlantean/Lemurian conflict in the battle of the masculine versus feminine energies and in the male versus female social roles, there is an East/West conflict around communal consciousness versus individuality . It would be very useful for the yellow race to learn to integrate more experience and celebration of individuality. They also could learn how to embrace their unique emotional bodies to not compete with but rather further compliment what they have achieved through their dynamic communal culture.

## The White Race

The white race includes Europeans, Russians, Arabs, Persians, Turks, most Jews[16], and the many nationalities of Caucasus region and the central Asian plains east of the Caspian Sea, as well as descendants of all these peoples in the Americas. The Pakistani are a hybrid between the white and brown races. Spiritually, they vibrate closer to the white race.

The majority of the white race came to Earth from Meldek, a planet that existed between Mars and Jupiter which destroyed itself in a nuclear war (thus creating the asteroid belt). Other soul energies of the white race came from the Orion and Pleiadian systems. These soul groups came to Earth with a highly developed mental body and a highly underdeveloped emotional body. The Cosmic history of the white race has been to continually excel in technology, science, warfare and intellect while denying the emotional and intuitive capacities. Souls incarnate in the white race consciousness to meet this extreme imbalance and to learn to acknowledge and experience the emotional body to heal this mentally aggressive pattern that has caused the physical destruction of so many of their previous home planets.

The white race is the most intellectual of the five races. This does not mean that the white race is more intelligent, only that it attaches its identity more to the intellect than any of the other races. As the white race works out its karma — which is to balance its over-emphasized intellect with an equal measure of emotional embodiment — then its scientific and technologically inventive brilliance can bring upliftment and fulfillment to all of humanity instead of war, imperialism and suppression of the other races.

---

16 There exists a substantial body of Ethiopian black Jews.

It is important to acknowledge the beneficial gifts the white race has made in scientific achievements, literature, music, art, exploration and discovery as well as instilling a deep sense of pioneering individualism and enthusiastic creativity to the whole of human consciousness. The challenge is their willingness to blend emotions and Earth connections from the other racial experiences as well as the intellectual and creative experiences of all groups to balance their tendencies towards over-intellectualism, intolerance and aggressive control.

## Racial & Religious Mirroring

When looking at the racial karmas, it becomes evident why certain races choose to experience certain religions. Many Orientals vibrate towards Buddhism, using this belief system to deny personal desires and emotions. This is in reality to support their need for security in unified consciousness by suppressing individual feelings and needs. The brown races' magnetism towards Hinduism and Goddess religions reflects their commitment to Mother Earth and all Her facets through the nature spirits. But it also reflects the fragmentation that has resulted from the over-commitment to Earth to the point of severely denying their own masculine energy and personal emotional needs. And certainly, the victimization by the imbalanced masculine energy of the white race is clearly reflected in the aggressive take-over of their culture by the Christian and Muslim religions. Both Christianity and Islam aggressively reject feminine energy. This abusive imbalanced masculine energy of the white race serves as a reflection to the brown and black races of their denial of masculine energy.

The black race has been enslaved by many races, including their own, as a reflection of the victimhood and sense of inferiority that *they judge upon themselves*, and which they brought with them to this planet from the Sirian system. Again, we say that this inferiority has no basis in reality. It is a self-judgment that they simply brought with them to this planet to continue healing. Because they have denied their own sense of equality, they magnetized the subjugation of the other races, including cultures of their own group consciousness.

What enslaved the black race more than the slavery itself was their forced conversion by their white masters to Christianity. This enslaved them far more cruelly than their actual experience as slaves. Christianity is a Piscean Age religion, addicted to belief as a way to paradise. It teaches you that the good must suffer on Earth and receive the rewards in an afterlife by a totally loving God — but only if you believe the "right" way. Nothing can enslave a soul more heartlessly than holding to this belief. Much of the blacks' projected blame and resentment towards other races is now being acted out in a highly aggressive Muslim and fundamentalist Christian experience. The black race has much self-owning and healing to do around this.

The white race has been predominately Judeo-Christian, and later Muslim, which are all highly intellectual and in severe denial of the feminine energies and the emotional body. Lately there has been a mass exodus of the white consciousness into Buddhism, *thinking* it is becoming more loving and gentle within Buddhism when in fact, this is just a further avoidance of their emotional ownership. The white race is so addicted to intellectual belief system that they have scavenged the planet with missionaries and capitalism to force everyone else to accept their belief system out of a severe denial and fear of emotional self-ownership. The white race has an enormous karmic challenge to clean up this aggressively projected mess and start taking ownership of its emotional needs.

Everyone incarnates into all races and nationalities to embody and experience every facet and variation of the karmic responsibility in order to learn how to own and be themselves one hundred per cent. Besides the fact that prejudice is damaging in its unlovingness, it is also a waste of time because we must incarnate as all races and nationalities. We are therefore judging, condemning and punishing ourselves in our other facets of experience when we stubbornly insist on playing this prejudicial game.

## Unresolved Atlantean Karma

Although unresolved Atlantean karma permeates every soul on the planet, there are seven nations that most aggressively act out the Atlantean karma for the rest of the world. These seven countries are: United States of America, Russia, Sweden, France, Germany, Great Britain and Australia. These seven countries magnetize most powerfully those souls with the heaviest unfinished Atlantean memories and issues to act out, to come to an inner emotional ownership for healing.

These countries have the greatest influence on all the other countries in the world in how they try to influence, dominate and control everyone else as a projection of their denied emotional bodies and rejected feminine energies.

Especially Russia and the Nordic countries of Denmark, Norway, Sweden, Finland and Iceland act out a mental idealism of a perfect society that tries to make everyone the same to the severe denial and destruction of the individual soul and the emotional body.

There is much these countries have to teach other countries about the positive dynamics of communal living and consideration. We feel that Russia and the Nordic countries are imbalanced in an idealism that, since it is not appropriately balanced with sufficient feminine/emotional embodiment, there is much mental coldness, fear and cultural control that is highly destructive to the souls living within those soul groups.

## Canada & New Zealand

Canada and New Zealand are two countries that are presently achieving a healthier integration and balance of the masculine and feminine energies that the seven Atlantean countries stubbornly continue to resist. "The Atlantean Seven" would have much to learn from Canada and New Zealand if they could get off their arrogantly intellectual high horses and graciously learn from the more gentle humanism of these two countries.

At the same time, Canada and New Zealand need to integrate more trust and emotional embodiment of their masculine energy and not perceive themselves as the "little brothers"[17] to the seven Atlantean countries.

[17] Feeling inferior.

## Latin American & Mediterranean Countries

The Latin American and Mediterranean countries are allowing themselves a greater expression of their emotional bodies. They do so however with a severely imbalanced denial of the intellectual bodies. They feel and express their emotions but tend to project them willy-nilly without more fully taking conscious responsibility to own what they are creating and reflecting from within themselves. The Latin American and Mediterranean countries are still a bit addicted to being victims of the "Atlantean Seven" and need to heal their own inferiority complexes instead of merely blaming them upon others. While they possess tremendous heart energy that Earth desperately needs, the primary karmic lesson these national soul groups are evolving toward at this time is a deeper trust in their own sense of worth.

It is vitally important that all races embody a higher conscious acknowledgment and celebration of the feminine energy and its equal power with the masculine. All races and nationalities need to recognize that they mirror their denial of self-love to one another and project the victim/victimizer game upon one another. Everybody is caught up in the great dance of avoiding self-creativity and self-ownership. Let us all come from the deepest attunement of our hearts which recognizes all souls as one and the same regardless of sex, religion, race, or nationality.

# Appendix I
# Chakras

There are chakras of the body as well as chakras on the Earth. We will first describe the body chakras, followed by the Earth chakras.

## Base Chakra

This is often referred to as the survival chakra, since this is the first manifestation of the life force in the physical body. We like to think of it as the foundation chakra. The rest of the body and the other chakras are supported by this foundation. The symbol for the base chakra is the square and the color is red. The Universal energies rise up the spinal column from the first and second chakras. This energy is called *Kundalini* or *Chi*.

A lack of optimal functioning in this chakra manifests in some people as fatigue. In other people, it manifests as self-centered, arrogant behavior. They may feel that the way to get what they want is to use *force*. This simply means that the person experiences fear in connecting fully to God, or the Divine Energies. They are often afraid for their own survival. They may not be able to concentrate on anything except making money, protecting their home, sleeping and getting enough to eat and drink.

A person with a weak base chakra may be someone who "lives in their head," is spaced out, or is only interested in the creative arts but is not very practical. Remember that we all need to use both sides of our brain, and we need to also be grounded. When we are grounded, we have a good connection to planet Earth. When we have a good, strong connection to the Earth, we have a pathway to send disharmonious vibrations out of our physical and subtle bodies. Grounding uses the same mechanism as the roots of trees to discharge energies which are not necessary. Trees and the Earth use our waste product of metabolism — carbon dioxide — and return oxygen to us. Mother Earth takes the disharmonious, "used" energies (like old ideas that no longer serve our vision or formerly repressed emotions), and we are given fresh energies from Father Sky, or God, which come in through the crown chakra.

The endocrine glands[18] associated with the base chakra are the adrenal glands. These are responsible for producing hormones, most importantly adrenaline. Remember that the base chakra is also called the survival chakra. When we feel that our survival is threatened, the adrenal glands will pump our bodies full of adrenaline and place us in a state of fight or flight readiness. Caffeine also stimulates the secretion of adrenaline. If a person is mostly operating out of the base chakra, the adrenal glands are usually weakened from abuse (over-stimulation). The person may drink a lot of caffeine-containing substances or other stimulant drugs in the attempt to recharge. Other areas of the body related to this chakra include the skin, kidneys and urinary bladder.

The essential oils and oil blends of Cedarwood, Grounding, Harmony, Juniper, Sacred Mountain (and all

[18] Endocrine glands are glands that secrete substances, e.g. hormones, into the body, for example into the blood stream or cerebrospinal fluid. This as opposed to exocrine glands that secrete substances to the outside of the body, for example onto the skin or into the stomach or intestines. (The inside of the gastrointestinal tract is, physiologically speaking, outside of the body.) The pancreas is both an endocrine and an exocrine gland.

conifer oils), Sage, Valerian and Valor may be of assistance in supporting and strengthening the first (base) chakra.

## Creative Chakra

This chakra is generally called the sexual chakra, possibly because the endocrine glands associated with this chakra are the reproductive glands. The symbol of the second chakra is the triangle and its color is orange. We feel the term, "creative chakra" better suits this chakra, since sexual activity is only one aspect of creativity. Other terms that are used are "navel chakra" and "relationship chakra."

The way to create from this chakra is to allow the foundation energies from the first chakra to rise up to the level of this chakra. We now have support, as the first chakra energies meet and merge with the second chakra energies for creation to take place. Note that the manifestation of this creation takes place at the level of the throat chakra.

When the creative chakra is not functioning optimally, one may experience challenges in the reproductive system — ovaries, uterus, fallopian tubes, prostate, testicles and penis. Blockages in this chakra also take the form of not creating what we desire. Or we may be very creative and have a lot of energy in this area, but we aren't allowing this energy to rise to the level of the throat chakra for it to manifest.

The second chakra is also the chakra out of which we build personal intimate relationships with other people. It is the seat of our sexual energy, our life force, prana, chi, or whatever term we choose to use, and our sexuality is the ultimate way in which we express ourselves in an intimate relationship. The sexuality doesn't have to be expressed physically for there to be a flow of sexual energy passing between two people's relationship/sexual chakras and bond them in an intimate relationship. A deep friendship is enough, even between two heterosexual people of the same sex. So an imbalanced second chakra will create problems with any type of intimate relationships. This can express itself as aloofness, erratic behavior and lack of dependability in relationships, as well as compulsive sex addiction.

Essential oils and oil blends of Bergamot, Clary Sage, Dragon Time, Gentle Baby, Geranium, Harmony, Inner Child, Joy, Lavender, Mister, Nutmeg, Patchouly, SARA and Tangerine may be of assistance in supporting and strengthening the second (creative) chakra.

## Solar Plexus

This is the power seat of the emotional body. The symbol is the circle and its color is yellow. Some call it the chakra of will power. It is the place through which we interact with the world. If one's body carries excess fat around the abdomen, this can signify that this person desires to symbolize a large power center out of which to operate in the world. This could be due to a feeling of lack or weakness. If this chakra is functioning well, people trust themselves to let their power flow. They feel and express their power and use it to create by combining with the energies of the first two chakras. This chakra is also associated with the great pleasure that comes from deeply knowing one's unique place within the Universe and thus, one feels empowered.

When the solar plexus is not functioning optimally, the person often stores unexpressed power inside. Unexpressed power can turn into anger or rage, depending on how long the energy has been denied expression. This can manifest as excess fat or excessive thinness around this chakra, in the belly. Or, it can manifest as disease in the intestines. When this chakra is not functioning well, people often do not trust the Universe or themselves. They do not feel empowered. They don't feel there is any place or purpose for them in the world. They may have a lot of anger due to not being in touch with how to utilize their power. Depending on which way the individual chooses to take this imbalance, he or she may withdraw from the world to become a gray and incognito persona, become a powerless victim and martyr of "random and meaningless" events, or he/she may overcompensate and become a great abuser of power — a tyrant — in the fear of being powerless.

A person with an imbalanced Solar Plexus Chakra is not letting the emotional energies of the lower three chakras flow through his or her Solar Plexus to meet with the mental energies of the upper chakras at the level of the heart. A block at the solar plexus can be seen in a person's aura as a black band at the level of the diaphragm. In essence, these people don't fully embrace their emotions, and thus they don't empower their emotions, which in turn would empower themselves.

The endocrine gland associated with this chakra is the pancreas which produces insulin. Insulin assists glucose — the main fuel for the body — in reaching its destination. On a spiritual level, this is symbolic of being empowered with Divine energy. The liver, gall bladder and stomach are also associated with the solar plexus chakra.

People with unexpressed energies in this chakra may drink a lot of alcohol, eat a lot of sugar or use drugs (recreational or prescription). These activities could create hypoglycemia, diabetes or drug addiction. We consider all substances a person abuses as drugs to cover up the pain of holding down this expression. If one abuses sugar, then sugar is their drug. We feel a person uses drugs to cover up the fact that they really feel insecure and inadequate. This insecurity is a judgment that causes denial and separation in the body which causes a lack of fully connecting to the Divine Energies. Yes, there are many areas to investigate in addictions. These are discussed in Dr. Marcy Foley's books, *Integrating Your Wholeness* and *Embraced by the Essence.*

What is needed in all cases of substance abuse is to free up the solar plexus so a person can feel their Divine power. When this chakra is unblocked, the energy can rise to the level of the heart chakra so people can feel their emotions and the love of the Universe. When you are grounded at your base chakra, you then use your life force to create with a loving intention, and then connect this to your personal power. The next step is to move this energy up to the heart chakra and to add the power from your emotional body into your life expression.

Essential oils and oil blends of Gentle Baby, Geranium, Grounding, Harmony, Inner Child, Lavender, Live with Passion, Patchouly, Sacred Mountain and SARA, may be of assistance in supporting and strengthening the third (solar plexus) chakra.

## Heart Chakra

The heart chakra is the gateway to the emotional body and is the chakra of giving and receiving love. Love is who you are. The symbol is the heart-shape and its colors are green and pink. The heart chakra is the balance between the upper three and the lower three chakras. When this chakra functions optimally, the person experiences unity with All That Is and finds it pleasurable and safe to give love to the self and others. When one is able to trust enough (allowing the energies to rise from the solar plexus chakra) to love oneself and to feel lovable, then one is also capable of giving and expressing love to others as well as receiving love from others.

Love is really the coming together and balance of one's masculine and feminine energies in one's heart. It is one's masculine mental energies in love with one's feminine emotional energies and one's feminine side in love with one's masculine side. A perfect balance between the feminine and masculine sides in an individual is extremely rare. In many people, these two aspects are actually at war with each other, rather than in love. Such people often don't even know what love really is, even though they may behave very "lovingly." They confuse guilt with love and perform "acts of love" for their parents, children, friends and others, believing that they do these things out of love when in fact they do them out of guilt. But because they've never experienced love within themselves for themselves, they have no way of knowing the difference between kindness out of love and kindness out of guilt.

When unexpressed energies are weighing down the heart chakra, the person may experience fear in giving love. Their fear is that if they give out love, there won't be enough love for them. Or perhaps the person with a heart chakra which is not optimally functioning can only give, and give, and give, thus depleting their energies, because they can't trust enough (solar plexus chakra) to receive love. These people may think of themselves as the Universal Mother/Nurturer type, whether or not this person is a male or a female. This type of imbalance also occurs in a person who is very withdrawn and may be able to interact with books, computers, and things of a mechanical nature, but not with people.

Blockage at the level of the heart chakra can manifest as a person who has heart disease — heart attack, stroke, or atherosclerosis, leading to by-pass surgery. Though because the heart chakra is a balancing influence, the lower three or upper three chakras are often the source of the dysfunction. The endocrine gland associated with the heart chakra is the thymus gland, part of the immune system. Thus, all kinds of problems associated with not keeping out disharmonious energy (such as disease) will occur if the heart chakra is repressed or contracted. The major illnesses of our time — AIDS, cancer and heart problems — all involve the heart chakra in connection with the lower chakras.

Associated problems with the heart chakra could occur in the respiratory tract, such as asthma, emphysema and bronchitis. All challenges in the respiratory tract are life-threatening because one cannot live longer than a few minutes without enough oxygen. Chronic health challenges associated with not taking in enough oxygen certainly make for a miserable way to live. Shallow breathing could represent a shallow life because one cannot experience the full love and joy that God intended for us if one cannot give and receive love. *What could be more life-threatening than to think or feel (even if it is not true) cut off from the Source of all love?* When one is able to unconditionally give and receive love, beginning with the ability to love oneself, life-threatening diseases will not be able to manifest because there is too high of a frequency for them to manifest.

Emotionally, there are many indications of a weak or imbalanced heart chakra, the obvious ones being expressions of heartlessness, cruelty, being emotionally cold and uncaring, being aloof or withdrawn. Less obvious indications are shame, embarrassment, smothering, being an over-caretaker of others or being guilt-ridden.

Essential oils and oil blends of Forgiveness, Gathering, Gentle Baby, Harmony, Hope, Inner Child, Joy, Lavender, Live With Passion, Orange, Present Time, SARA, Spikenard and White Angelica may be of assistance in supporting and strengthening the fourth (heart) chakra.

## Throat Chakra

This is the chakra of manifesting our creations from the second chakra. It is the power seat of the mental body. The symbol is the equilateral cross and its color is blue. When functioning optimally, this is where one takes responsibility for all that occurs in one's Universe. If this chakra does not function well, people act like victims or martyrs and blame others for what happens in their lives. The endocrine gland associated with this chakra is the thyroid gland, the energy switchboard of the body necessary for optimal growth and metabolism.

The throat chakra is also the chakra for all types of expression, not just verbal. Stuttering, difficulty finding the words to express oneself, being a "motor mouth", excessive or subdued body language can all be indications of an imbalanced throat chakra. Quietness may or may not be an indication of an imbalanced throat chakra. We live in a culture where being a good conversationalist is more or less expected of all of us. People may be quiet out of shyness or lack of verbal abilities, but they may also be so because they are at peace within themselves. They may just not feel pressured by the social and cultural expectations that make us always want to keep a conversation going just for the sake of making other people feel comfortable. Even with a well functioning throat chakra, some people enjoy talking and others don't. Neither are necessarily signs of a weak throat chakra, although both can be.

When energy is repressed in the throat chakra, it may manifest as a metabolic rate which is either too slow or too fast, producing a distortion in the optimum amount of body fat. It may manifest as not enough energy to do one's desired tasks. Or, there is unfocused energy which expresses itself as hyperactivity or nervousness. In either event, if this chakra is repressed or overly excited, people will have difficulties manifesting what they desire.

Signs to look for when this chakra is congested include a chronic cough, always clearing the throat, sore throat, laryngitis and neck problems (such as subluxated cervical vertebrae which don't hold an adjustment).

The secondary gland involved in the throat chakra is the parathyroid, which is responsible for calcium metabolism. Stored energy or a depletion of energy in the throat chakra could take the form of bone abnormalities, such as osteoporosis, or excess calcification in any of the bones. Associated healing challenges could also occur in the ears with infections or hearing trouble. The sinuses are also involved and could manifest congestion or infection if the throat chakra is not happy.

Essential oils and oil blends of Blue (German) Chamomile, Dream Catcher, Harmony, Live with Passion, Magnify Your Purpose, Motivation, 3 Wise Men, Release, and SARA may be of assistance in supporting and strengthening the fifth chakra.

## Brow Chakra

This chakra is the psychic or intuitive center, which provides the capacity to visualize and optimally work with the energies of the Universe. The brow chakra could also be called the center of introspection — the gateway to the mental body — where consciousness probes into itself. The third dimensional symbol is the crescent and its color is indigo, which is a deep blue color with just a hint of red in it. When this chakra functions well, the person easily taps into their intuition, their mental abilities, and is well aware of their ideas. When repressed, the person may experience mental frustration, not being able to bring their ideas to their conscious awareness or not being able to bring their ideas into fruition. This malfunction could create a situation where a person lacks intuition and common sense.

While the throat chakra is the chakra of manifestation in the sense that it is the center of expression and "taking action," the brow chakra also contains important energies related to manifestation. The brow chakra is the center of mental clarity, which is necessary in order to bring our thoughts and ideas into fruition — or manifestation — in a practical, working manner.

The endocrine gland associated with the brow chakra is the pituitary, the master gland in the body which regulates all the others. If there isn't sufficient energy in the adrenals, ovaries, pancreas, thymus, thyroid and parathyroid, the pituitary must work overtime, thus exhausting one's mental energy as well as one's energy for creativity and manifestation.

Repressed energies in the brow chakra can affect the lower brain and eyes. Remember, the physical eyes are symbolic of the status of the spiritual eyes. Needing corrective support for the eyes means attunement to the spiritual eyes may need to be stronger. If there is stagnation or over-stimulation and aberrations in the mental body, this may result in congestion in the brain, giving rise to such conditions as A.D.D. and Alzheimer's disease.

Essential oils and oil blends of Awaken, Clarity, Frankincense, Galbanum, Harmony, Inspiration, Magnify Your Purpose, Motivation, Present Time, Release, Sandalwood, Spikenard, Surrender and 3 Wise Men may be of assistance in supporting and strengthening the sixth chakra.

## Crown Chakra

This is the spiritual center, the connection to the wholeness of oneself. It's symbol is the four-leaf-clover or the thousand petaled lotus flower. It's color is purple or violet. When the crown chakra functions optimally, the person feels whole, complete, and trusts enough to invite the inner God to co-create. When repressed, the person often feels cut off from God, does not realize their connection to All That Is and denies the unity present in nature. The person feels everything has to be scientifically proven and negates the mystical and magical aspects of the metaphysical or the unseen world.

The brow and the crown chakras are both seats of intuitive knowledge that in some cases is received from other planes of existence. When this knowledge comes through the brow chakra, it is often more direct in the form of images, words or strong feelings. People with these abilities are called clairvoyant, clairaudient, or clairsentient. If the same intuitive knowledge comes by way of the crown chakra, it is usually in the form of an inexplicable "knowing." This is similar to clairsentience but is more vague with less feelings associated with it.

The endocrine gland associated with the crown chakra is the pineal gland. The pineal gland is a photo receptor[19] and is involved in the production of the hormones melatonin, serotonin and other important compounds in the body. Repressed energies in this chakra manifest as upper brain congestion (possibly involving neurological disease), improper regulation of certain endocrine glands and skin pigmentation problems.

Essential oils and oil blends of Awaken, Clarity, Dream Catcher, Frankincense, Galbanum, Harmony, Humility, Inspiration, Magnify Your Purpose, Motivation, Release, Sandalwood, Surrender, 3 Wise Men and Spikenard may be of assistance in supporting and strengthening the seventh chakra.

[19] A photoreceptor is something which detects light.

# Earth's Chakra Points

Just as the body has chakras, so does the Earth. Chakras receive and ground vibratory energies from higher dimensions of this and other Universes as well as emanate these energies across the planet, influencing all life existing near these chakra points. To physically visit Earth's chakra points can powerfully catalyze the healing of issues within us that are related to that particular chakra. The shift from the Age of Pisces to the Age of Aquarius takes place over a 25 year period from 1987 to 2012.

| **Piscean Age (Previous 2,000 Years)** | | |
|---|---|---|
| **Emanating Color** | **Chakra** | **Location** |
| Red | Root | India |
| Orange | Creative | Tibet |
| Yellow | Solar Plexus | Sedona, AZ, U.S.A. |
| Green, Pink | Heart | Maui, Hawaii, U.S.A. |
| Blue | Throat | Front Range of U.S. Rocky Mountains |
| Indigo | Third Eye | British Isles |
| Purple, Violet | Crown | Mt. Shasta, CA, U.S.A. |

| Aquarian Age (Next 2,000 Years) | | |
|---|---|---|
| **Emanating Color** | **Chakra** | **Location** |
| Red | Root | India |
| Orange | Creative | Tibet |
| Yellow | Solar Plexus | Front Range of U.S. Rocky Mountains, from Albuquerque, NM to Boulder, CO |
| Green, Pink | Heart | Ayers Rock, Central Australia |
| Blue | Throat | Central Norway and Sweden |
| Indigo | Third Eye | British Isles |
| Purple, Violet | Crown | Sedona, AZ, U.S.A. |

## Root and Creative Chakras

Historically, early recorded human life occurred in the land between the Tigris and Euphrates Rivers in the Middle East, an area influenced by the Source (Root) and Creative

Chakras. World karmic issues continue to erupt in this region and east of it as these two chakras remain in India and Tibet, birthplaces of several of the primary religions and cultures of Earth. The creative roots to almost everything that exists today can be historically traced to this area of the world, the Middle East, India and the Far East.

## Solar Plexus Chakra

The large number of chakra points in the United States during the Age of Pisces reveal the energies that magnetized Old World Europeans, Africans and Asians to the Americas as the next step in human evolution.

Especially in the past 100 years, a predominance of spiritual studies, books, techniques and teachers have come out of America. The Solar Plexus, Throat and Crown Chakras of the Piscean Age drew explorers and immigrants to the Americas during the past 1,000 years. The Solar Plexus and Crown Chakras remain in the United States during the Aquarian Age, in shifted locations, as the dominating influence of this country will continue to escalate.

The Solar Plexus Chakra stimulates the emotional body, and especially the most suppressed emotional memories. It is worth noting that since this chakra has shifted to the Front Range of the Rocky Mountains, there has been an increase in the shootings and violence there (for example, the Columbine High School shootings in Littleton, Colorado). United States is a group consciousness heavy on emotional suppression, covered up with mental over-activity. The longer and deeper the emotional suppression, the greater the violent experiences needed to force the energies to the conscious surface.

## Heart Chakra

The Heart Chakra is now at Ayers Rock in the central outback of Australia, the heart center of what was once feminine-dominated Lemuria. This is no coincidence as the Aquarian Age ushers in the return of the Lemurian tradition of honoring the Goddess.

## Throat Chakra

The Throat Chakra has shifted in the Aquarian Age to central Norway and Sweden. Centuries ago, Nostradamus predicted that "the Light will come from the North."[20] This chakra point is catalyzing the reawakening souls who lived as the spiritual teachers and pioneers known as the Cathars, primarily in southern France in the 11th-14th centuries. The Cathars attempted to bring Europe out of the Dark Ages of church-controlled thought, but were killed *en masse* (usually burned at the stake) for daring to question the rigid, intolerant control of the church.

Most of these souls fled to Scandinavia for their current day incarnation, thinking they would be safe hiding away in that far corner of the world. But we cannot outsmart the Universe. The Throat Chakra energies now manifesting there challenges these souls to confront and own their fears in order to resurrect their long-suppressed knowledge and power.

---

[20] Nostradamus himself reincarnated in Scandinavia in the 17th century as the Swedish scientist, mystic and philosopher Emanuel Swedenborg. The church founded by Swedenborg's followers on his doctrines – the Church of the New Jerusalem – still to this day has followers in the United States.

## Third Eye/Brow Chakra

For the past 2,000 years the British Isles has been the arena of tremendous spiritual energy, culture and archetypal history. England has always been extremely intellectual, but with a very deep and profound spiritual tradition. This is reflected in its continuance as the Brow Chakra since the Piscean Age. The British Isles are remnants of Atlantis, holding on to the masculine and intellectually dominated Atlantean culture.

## Crown Chakra

Much of the southwestern United States was under water when Lemuria and Atlantis existed. Sedona was then a holy island of spiritual initiation at different times to both of those cultures. Hence, in the past 2,000 years it has held the Solar Plexus, and now the Crown Chakra points. Sedona is holy to many Native American tribes with ties to either Atlantean or Lemurian culture.

# Appendix II
# Therapies for Self-Healing

## Giving Ourselves Permission to Heal

Some of us need to give ourselves permission to heal, enjoy and create our lives the way that we choose for them to be. We are our own ultimate authority figures. We are our own saviors. No one can do this for us. It is so often true that most people want things to be different in their lives yet have not felt it was possible to have anything different. They feel powerless to change and thus feel stuck, hopeless or victimized. Only when we see our patterns and issues for what they are can we then accept them and embrace them from the depths of our beings. We will then have the greatest chance to change.

## Reclaiming Our True Power

It is time to reclaim our full power as the Gods and Goddesses we indeed are! This may sound like a radical or even blasphemous attitude, yet it is true. We have inherent within our birthright all the emotions, powers and abilities of Mother/Father God. All of us have abused power in other life experiences and have felt guilty, ashamed, bad and wrong because of this. We sought to punish and blame ourselves for this misuse of power, which then took the form of choosing lifetimes where someone else held "power" over us even though it was we who gave our power away and chose those experiences. For some of us, it was appropriate to live seemingly as victims and martyrs for the experience that that would give us. Perhaps we needed to feel our anger and rage strongly enough to then choose to be in our power without abusing it.

Forgive and accept yourself for not knowing how to use power in true unconditional love in the past. Choose to use your full power now. Choose to trust yourself to act in love, the love that you really are. Choose to stop rejecting, blaming and judging yourself for your past "mistakes." Realize that there were no mistakes. We needed to play out certain roles to learn what we needed to learn. We are where we are now, with our present consciousness, because of experiences we had in other incarnations. Honor that whatever you did — no matter what seemingly "sordid" things they were — you gained precious experiences to bring you to this moment of now. Claim your power and use it in love, with all the wisdom of your being. Honor the truth that the ultimate lesson is to learn that power is abused only because of lack of self-love.

Give yourself permission to discover and own your patterns, issues and what your body communicates to you. Give yourself permission to be in your power, to love, honor and respect yourself. *We make these commitments to others when we get married, and it is time to extend this commitment to ourselves in these same ways*. Then, we live our own honor codes and take personal responsibility for everything, for all experiences in our lives.

## Healing Modalities

After providing information on diseases, disorders, parts of the bodies and their symbolic meanings, what follows is a list of therapies that can help you in working on a practical level with the physical, emotional, mental and spiritual healing of the conditions you experience in your own life. It is not a complete list, and we will add here that the authors neither promote nor negate any therapies listed here. We list our truths concerning them for your own education in discerning how you choose to utilize these tools to heal yourself.

## Accupuncture/Accupressure Therapy

The application of needles to pressure points upon the body is an ancient healing practice derived from the Orient. This is a tremendously powerful healing tool to achieve relief from pain; alleviation of inflammation in muscles, joints, ligaments, tendons and the nervous system; harmonizing and balancing the energy meridians that flow throughout the body; balancing and cleansing toxins, bacteria and parasites from organs, the lymph system and the blood; alleviation of fever; and just about anything else you can think of.

What distinguishes Accupuncture from Accupressure is that Accupuncture uses needles[21] while Accupressure applies stimulation to the pressure points using the thumb or fingers. This is an especially excellent therapy to incorporate with other body treatments or emotional processing

[21] There is now Accupuncture that uses laser beams.

therapies. The use of therapeutic quality essential oils provides a wonderful addition to Accupuncture or Accupressure.

## Aromatherapy

Aromatherapy is the art and science of the use of therapeutic quality essential oils. The practice of Aromatherapy varies from country to country. In England it is often considered a form of massage where essential oils are rubbed into the body. In Germany, it is primarily just smelling the oils. In France the oils are most often ingested, snorted through the nose, as well as rubbed on the body. In America, all forms are used, with the ingestion of oils the least common.

The sense of smell is a very powerful way to bring to the surface and clear out blocked emotional memories. Essential oils exude scents that in themselves can have immediate and powerful healing results. There are also chemical constituents within the oils that penetrate the cellular walls to break down blockages and stimulate purifying healing and energetic movement that accelerates healing on all levels simultaneously.

Aromatherapy has gotten to be one of the new "buzz" words these days, which has resulted in the fact that the therapeutic quality of the work is often greatly compromised. The true practice of Aromatherapy involves only the highest quality essential oils — processed properly with low temperature and pressure — which come from plants, roots, tree bark or flowers that are grown organically without chemical pesticides or fertilizers. The oils are not extracted with chemicals or "extended" with chemical fillers. However, since most Americans don't know the difference, shampoo companies put some mixture of 95% synthetic "essential oils" mixed with 5% "pure" essential oils and call it an Aromatherapy shampoo. This is indeed unfortunate, as the true practice of Aromatherapy is one of the most beautiful forms of healing that exist today. This is the oldest recorded form of medicine known on this planet. If this therapy appeals to you, you must be very discerning in the oils you select as well as the therapist you choose to assist you.

## Art Healing Therapy

Life is a physical reflection of symbolic communications from the Universe. Art is a creative expression that requires the harmonious integration of our masculine and feminine energies so that we may create and express a symbolic picture of our thoughts and feelings. Art has been a powerful healing tool for centuries as it allows us to connect to the depths of our hidden knowledge, emotional feelings, healing needs and power potentials.

The Art Healing therapist will suggest a theme for the individuals to meditate upon for a few moments and connect with as deeply and emotionally within themselves as possible. These themes could include how they feel about their mother, their father, their inner child, their greatest frustration, their greatest rage, their work, a relationship, or any other aspect of their lives. A life-size piece of paper is taped on a hard, solid wall. Using water-based colors, the individual does not use a paintbrush but rather applies the paints directly onto the paper with their hands. It is not necessary to draw actual pictures. Rather, the individual expresses through the paints on their hands whatever feelings come up about the theme the therapist suggests to them. Sometimes there are pictures and sometimes it is just shapes and forms and splashes of color. The point is to express with the whole body the feelings going on inside and use the colors on the hands to express symbolically on the paper what goes on inside.

When the person is done, they then step back and look at the painting, saying to themselves that what they have created is a direct expression of what goes on inside of them. They are then asked what emotions come up when they realize and accept this truth of what they have created. Then they're asked to express emotionally with words, sounds or physical movement the emotions that come up as they look at the picture they have created. This allows a tremendously supportive environment to act out any emotions that need to be expressed, which are not being projected to any other individual. Sometimes a person may cry, scream, laugh, sing, overtone, spit, yell or even tear up the paper and stomp on it and throw it in all directions. Some individuals have been known to comfort the painting as a way of comforting themselves, and may hug and caress it or cry against it. Others may rant and rave and rage at it to vent all the suppressed and unresolved emotions that are being allowed to be felt and expressed and are safely projected onto the picture, and not onto any individual.

This therapy can be done one-on-one with the therapist, and other times a therapist may have two, three, or four individuals doing a therapeutic session together. When there is more than one individual in a session, each person takes turns going into the paintings of the other individual(s) to share what emotions come up in them being mirrored by the other person's painting. They do not judge or criticize the other pictures, nor do they say what the picture means for the other creator. Instead, they only express what the other person's painting mirrors to them about their own emotions. This teaches people to feel safe expressing their creativity and emotions to others, and how to express what they feel in another person's work in a way that does not project judgment or blame onto another. It also teaches people to listen to others sharing their emotions and process and seeing that this is not a judgmental projection or threat to themselves. In this way, people learn how to support one another in a sharing process that has no projected judgment, blame, or expectation onto any other individual.

## Aura/Polarity Balancing Therapy

This is an energy emanation which is channeled through the practitioner. The hands are held in different patterns above the body to restore a properly balanced flow of energy within the aura or through the body. This technique is very regenerating in and of itself. It also works tremendously well in association with other body treatments or emotional processing therapies.

## Chiropractic Care

Chiropractic care involves the entire body, not just the spine. It involves bringing into alignment all the joints, tendons and connective tissues in the body. Certainly there is a tremendous amount of attention given to the spine, where we suppress much fear and resistance towards our chosen paths. Because the kundalini energy travels up and down the spine connecting and integrating the energies of all our major chakras, spinal alignment is extremely important, especially in how that alignment integrates with the totality of the physical body.

A great amount of past-life physical abuse and damages (caused in wars, accidents, diseases, and natural catastrophes) are stored in the spine, and particularly in and between the shoulder blades. Chiropractic care, especially when incorporated with massage, Aromatherapy, or any other forms of bodywork or energy manipulation, will assist tremendously in healing these past-life damages stored as energy or other physical blockages in the body.

## Creative Body Movement

Under this category we include dance, sacred dance, yoga, T'ai Ch'i, Chigon,[22] any spontaneous and creative body movement, and the martial arts. What differentiates sacred dance from other dances is that sacred dance is based on the old folk dances but is performed with conscious spiritual meanings expressed through each step. Sacred dance and spontaneous creative movement have been used across the centuries for Earth healing and even to control the weather and clear away pollution and Earthbound spirits clinging to the physical plane in areas of wars

[22] A technique very similar to T'ai Ch'i.

or natural catastrophes. There are many, many courses available in all these forms of dance and body movements. Any and all of these can have a profound impact on grounding and centering oneself in the body, and clearing out physical as well as emotional blockages.

## Dream Counseling Therapy

Dreams are our most direct communication with our Higher Selves. In the dream state, we experience through a highly sophisticated visual symbology a continuing processing of our karmic issues, emotional denials, fears, goals, possibilities and potentials. The symbolic language that is our dreams is created by each of us through our Higher Selves to promote acceleration of our conscious development, as well as offering continual growth and development, and deep emotional ownership and healing.

A dream counseling therapist can assist an individual in developing a greater conscious awareness of dreams as well as discovering their own unique dream symbolic language in order to derive the highest potential of learning and healing from their dreams.

We are first presented in our dreams with our unresolved lessons and possibilities. What we continue to ignore or deny (consciously or unconsciously) in our dreams then projects out and manifests as experiences in our external, awake life. If we then continue to avoid or deny the mirroring in our everyday lives, the issues manifest as disorders and diseases in the body. Working as deeply as possible with our dreams allows us the opportunity to not only accelerate our spiritual development and inner healing but also results in less of a need to create external or bodily experiences to act out what can be understood, felt, owned and accomplished through dream work. Dream journals and lucid dream awareness are some of the tools the therapist can work with as the dreamer explores the path of dream symbols and their impact on every level of our lives.

## Gestalt Therapy

This is an emotional therapeutic process in which some physical object such as a chair, a pillow, a picture or any other inanimate object is chosen as a symbolic representation of the focus of our emotional processing. We imagine the object to be a person, event or issue onto which we express all our emotional feelings. This allows a safe environment to project emotions as fully as possible to come into as complete an expression as possible of the emotions that need to be expressed and transformed. This is especially good for individuals who do not yet feel safe to interact with other individuals in an emotional healing process.

## Journal Work

If you choose to do some quiet healing work by yourself, working in your own journal is very powerful. You will be amazed at the answers you discover within you when you do this type of work.

You may work on your computer, write in a bound empty book or simply a spiral notebook. Do whatever is comfortable for you. You may simply write down your feelings. It's your journal, so you can be as messy or neat as choose to be. Write two or three lines high to express your anger and rage if that does it for you. Take one whole page and write, "I feel SO ANGRY!" (*or whatever you are feeling.*)

You can also draw a line vertically down the page and voice dialogue with yourself. Some have learned to channel their inner voice, or their Higher Self, this way. You may get to some really deep core issues by having a conversation with that "little voice" within you.

If you want to know your state of consciousness and where you are in your life process, take a piece of paper and write down the major people in your life. Start with your parents, brothers, sisters and significant others in your life. Later you can list friends, co-workers, neighbors and others. What do you like or dislike about these people? How do you feel around these people? It is perfectly acceptable to say you hate someone or hate certain qualities in people, your community and your world so long as you don't project this hatred on to others. We get to own our hatred as a part of Emotional Ownership. It is time to stop denying that which we hate, fear and have rage about so we can reclaim those lost emotions.

The next step is to find those qualities in us and own them. This is how we take responsibility for them as parts of us. The qualities we react strongly to in others may not be there to the same degree or in the exact same way in us, but those qualities in other people mirror something to us about us, or those people would not be in our lives.

If we don't like the relationships we have with others, we can take Emotional Ownership of these qualities within us and choose to change and transform anything we desire. Once we change, the people will either act out different roles in our lives or they will leave our lives. This is Universal Law.

## Kinesiology

This technique is a wonderful re-direction of energy flow to harmonize and balance the spine and extremities, energy meridians, the brain and much more throughout the body. It uses a technique called muscle testing which allows a direct communication with the body to determine its needs, the cause and effect of disorders, and to determine whether the source of the disorder is on the physical, emotional, mental or spiritual levels. This is a great opportunity to develop a very direct communicative link with the body to determine the most direct causes of physical imbalances and the best therapies and nutrients the body requires to re-balance and heal itself. Many individuals have derived a deeper understanding and appreciation for the many levels of their consciousness and being, and how it all interconnects through the physical body, by using Kinesiology.

There are many varieties of Kinesiology, such as Applied Kinesiology, Clinical Kinesiology, as well as other "take-offs" which use muscle testing that is similar to Applied Kinesiology — such a the Chiropractic techniques T.B.M. (Total Body Modification) and N.E.T. (Neuro Emotional Technique) — to access what emotions are blocked, when they originated, and what parts of the body they affect. While N.E.T. practitioners feel they can make certain adjustments to the spine and rub a few points and all "negative" emotions will disappear, we do not feel this is truly the case. We feel the recipient still must take full Emotional Ownership and lovingly embrace and feel his or her previously suppressed emotions in order for complete healing to take place. However, the technique N.E.T. is still very valuable in discovering blocked emotions and neuro-emotional patterns.

## Massage & Rolfing

Massage has for centuries been one of the most important and powerful tools in physical balancing and healing as well as the integration of the emotional, mental and spiritual bodies. Because America is in such a poor state of emotional, mental and spiritual health, from its puritanical imprinting about sex and the physical body, many people here have a strong, fearful resistance to massage because they see the naked body as only sexual, and sexuality as dangerous, dirty and base.

In reality, massage is a loving and powerfully healing experience, allowing blocked energy to move freely through the body, and crystallized toxins to be broken down and cleared away. For some people, massage can be a unique experience of feeling a loving, healing touch that is not automatically sexual and dangerous. There are many types of massage which we won't go into here except one, which is less well known — Intuitive Massage.

In intuitive massage, the practitioner allows their hands to guide them to the places within the individual which require assistance. Many intuitive massage therapists work with closed eyes. The recipient has the opportunity to exercise their own intuitive feelings in order to magnetize to themselves someone with whom they can feel safe and who can get the energy moving and the blockages and judgments cleared out.

Rolfing is an extremely deep massage that restructures the connective tissue of the body. Because it is so deep and intense, it is too painful for many people. It can be a good therapeutic experience for people with exceptionally rigid and locked-up connective tissues resulting from severe emotional denial and resistance. A person who is very sensitive physically would in all probability not wish to choose this more intense form of bodywork. But it can be a wonderfully positive support to those who need that extra stimulation of the tissue to let go of the severe emotional resistance trapped within the hardened connective tissue.

## Meditation

This is the one of the most misunderstood and most highly abused therapies on the planet. Most people abuse meditation by trying to get *out* of the body to escape their emotions rather than to go fully *into* the body, and thus into the emotions. The point of meditation is *not* to get into a state of nothingness, but rather to achieve being totally in our Selves in full harmony with our bodies and emotions.

It is important to understand that sitting quietly is not the only kind of meditation. Listening to music, singing, overtoning, dancing, gardening, walking in nature, doing the dishes, or folding the laundry are all wonderful forms of meditation. The most common kind of meditation, however, involves sitting quietly and emptying the mind. For some people this works, and for others it doesn't. If this kind of quiet sitting doesn't do it for you, then try an active meditation that includes body movement or music or being in nature.

There are techniques, such as TM, which operate through mantras. Continuously repeating a mantra will on some people have the effect of keeping them restricted to their heads and out of their emotions. We will state, however, that for people who have an over-active and noisy mind, this can be an excellent technique to discipline the mind to calm down and be quiet.

In some cases there are instructors who charge hundreds of dollars for a personal mantra and tell you not to reveal it to others. Is this because they charge hundreds of dollars to give the same mantra to hundreds of people? We ask you to discern for yourself. If you feel drawn to practice this type of technique, we ask you to carefully feel your feelings in regards to who you work with and what kind of meditation you use.

## Mind Control & Positive Thinking Techniques

It is important to dedicate nurturing to the mental body as well as to the emotional body. Too much focus on the emotional body to the extent of ignoring the mental body can cause just as much damage as those who deny the emotional by over-focusing on the mental. Mind Control and any positive thinking techniques can achieve a temporary assistance in helping those who are addicted to negative thinking and negative expectation, or who do not know how to appropriately clear and focus the mind. We feel it is important to state that these mental therapies are helpful mainly in this particular way. Once the mental discipline and stopping of negative addiction is achieved, there must be an incorporation of emotional processing and ownership as well. If not, all that has been achieved in the mental therapy is likely to become a destructive imbalance of emotional denial.

Mind Control is not a positive thinking therapy. It is about disciplining the mental body to achieve appropriate clarity, focus, goals, and achievement of those goals. We include it with the positive thinking therapies only because they all have to do with the mental body. The mental body needs appropriate nurturing. However, we must be careful not to over-focus on the mental or the emotional to the exclusion of the other, or else we get caught in a whirlpool of creating one imbalanced denial upon another.

## Music & Sound Therapy

It has been said that music is the Divine language of the Universe. Music is a direct creative expression of the highest GodSelf through incarnate being.

Listen to music that is especially soothing and comforting to you, and allow yourself to feel the music flow through your body so that you feel yourself becoming inseparably one with the music. This will allow blocked emotions to come to the surface to be felt, expressed and let go of. It is helpful to give sound to the emotions being triggered to the surface by the music, whether through singing, groaning, chanting, overtoning, crying, laughing, screaming, or making whatever noises you need in order to express and allow the emotions to be felt and cleared.

Singing and overtoning are, in themselves, powerful tools to elicit suppressed emotions to the surface to be felt and cleared. Toning is simply making sounds that seem appropriate to the person. Overtoning is when you get two sounds to come out of your mouth at once, often in harmony. This is very beneficial in vibrating your pineal and pituitary glands. A Sound Therapist can show you how to do this.

In working with Sound Therapy yourself, you simply feel into an unresolved emotion or experience, open your mouth and let that be expressed. You will feel the energies move. Some sounds will be pleasant, and some will not. It doesn't matter what the sounds are. Just honor that you are expressing yourself. Toning is a very powerful form of getting movement and expression through your throat chakra.

Playing any musical instrument can also achieve the same results. It is important to not judge any emotions as good or bad, right or wrong, spiritual or unspiritual. The point is not to get rid of the emotions but rather to feel them and allow them to be expressed for what they need to teach us about our relationships to ourselves. Emotions reveal judgment, guilt, criticism, negative expectation, belief systems, and old vows that control our lives and cause the real pain. The emotions are simply symbolic messages to help us connect to the real issues within the emotions.

Stringed instruments, in particular, vibrate very strongly to the heart and solar plexus chakras. Of particular help in music therapy is to listen to music of harps, Celtic harps and violin concertos. We particularly recommend the Celtic harp music of Alan Stivell — Renaissance of the Celtic Harp — and the violin concertos of Bruch, Tchaikovsky, Beethoven, Mendelssohn, and Dvorak. Certainly, playing these musical instruments will also create enormous emotional movement and healing. Courses in singing and overtone chanting will help tremendously in freeing blocked emotions to be expressed, healed and released.

## Past-Life Regression Therapy

In the DNA in every cell of our bodies we carry our Akashic Records, which is the accumulative totality of all our lifetimes of experiences, thoughts, emotions, belief systems, etc. It is from this accumulative vibration that we choose and create each new incarnate experience. Unresolved lessons, denied or avoided emotional experiences, thoughts and belief systems all affect what we experience, choose and create in this moment.

A past-life regression therapist can, through hypnotic guidance, lead an individual to particular lifetime situations and memories that feed and control how we think, feel, believe, anticipate and perceive what is happening now. By allowing ourselves to embrace and accept what happened in another lifetime, and especially by honoring what we need to feel from that experience — and thereby accept the true deeper meaning of what the experience represented — a completion can occur in the here and now so that growth, healing and a more consciously loving and creative experience can evolve from here on. A therapeutic experience such as this can help teach us that nothing is right or wrong, good or bad, spiritual or unspiritual, but that everything is simply a learning experience. Resolving unfinished or denied memories, and especially allowing full emotional ownership and acceptance of these experiences, help to alleviate self-judgment, guilt, and punishing behavior in which most of us tend to remain caught up.

It is important to state here that one should be on guard to not become too caught up in reliving other lifetimes, or in specific details. It is too easy a trap to become lost in other lifetimes as a way to avoid being fully present in one's life here and now. Any tool, no matter how potentially positive and healing, can become distorted and destructive if one becomes too obsessive or addicted to it. It is not necessary to actually remember or relive specific details of another lifetime to achieve the ownership and healing that can be derived. Sometimes just the feeling surrounding the experience is sufficient to achieve the required clearing and healing.

There are several types of hypnotic therapies that can assist in alleviating destructive or addictive behaviors that may or may not include memories of past lives. One needs to feel an intuitive comfort with the integrity, consciousness, emotional and spiritual clarity of the therapist before committing to this type of therapy.

## Psychodrama Therapy

In this therapy, we take the next step from Gestalt Therapy, in which we project our emotions onto an external, inanimate object. In Psychodrama, a person chooses a real life event, a dream, or a situation that they feel is emotionally unresolved and which needs the healing of emotional completion. The individual having the Psychodrama chooses other people to act out however many roles are required for the issue to be acted out. The therapist asks questions about the event, as well as the characteristics and roles of all individuals involved. Then, through the therapist's questions, everyone acts out the situation described by the individual creating the Psychodrama. The therapist will repeatedly ask questions about what the individual feels from moment-to-moment, what happens next, why they feel the situation evolves as it does, and again, what they feel through each new development of the drama.

What is most unique about Psychodrama Therapy is that every so often, the therapist assigns all the characters to change roles so that all individuals get to experience the situation from every point of view, and get to express the emotions of every character involved. This allows the individual whose Psychodrama it is to see the event or situation they are working on resolving from all points of view, and to get in touch as deeply as possible with all the previously blocked emotions within themselves as well as being provoked, challenged and expanded by feeling and expressing the emotions of all characters involved.

Also in Psychodrama, once a situation is clearly and fully experienced and expressed from all points of view, the individual can then create their Psychodrama to act itself out in whatever kind of a finale that will give them the greatest emotional healing, support and sense of completion. Typical examples of Psychodramas that individuals create in this therapy are rape, incestual abuse, divorce, child custody, being fired from a job, and any situation that resulted in an emotional trauma due to unresolved conflict.

Psychodramas can also be created to act out dreams, with individuals playing all the roles in order to derive the deepest meanings from that dream. Many individuals have used Psychodrama to act out a past-life memory in order to discover the meaning that memory has for them in this present incarnation. Also, individuals who have unresolved grief or rage at the death of family or friends have used Psychodrama to communicate and express the emotions towards the individual who has died in order to come to an emotional healing and completion with the death. In a Psychodrama, there is a role reversal so that they then must play the role of the person who has passed on, and another individual is role playing them. This allows tremendously powerful layers of denied emotions and potential healing and learning to integrate into their consciousness and lives.

Still another way to use this therapy is to act out a Psychodrama with someone portraying cigarettes, alcohol, drugs, or any addiction so that the individual can communicate and emotionally express all the issues surrounding the addiction. Here again, several times during the Psychodrama, the other individual will portray them as they portray the addiction to bring them into even deeper emotional contact and understanding of the real reasons for the addiction and the highest lessons and healing to be derived from that addictive experience.

## Rebirthing/Connective Breathing

Breath is life. In the way we breathe, we reveal all the blockages and denials in our bodies. Rebirthing is a therapy that allows us to literally breathe into these blockages and denials to clear away that blocked energy and allow movement of emotion through the body. Connective breathing is powerful in breaking down mental resistance, to allow emotional expression to break through. We need to state here that there are unfortunately many rebirthers who are not sufficiently connected to their own Emotional Ownership, and therefore tend to maintain the rebirthing session on a mental level. It is important that an individual use intuitive feeling to discern a rebirther who shows themselves open to emotional feeling and processing. This way, the connective breathing will allow for emotional ownership and feeling rather than solely focusing on the mental thought processes. Don't be afraid to ask direct questions to the therapist about their beliefs and relationships to emotions to help you determine who feels right to assist you in this potentially powerful therapeutic experience.

## Reflexology

Every single part of the body has corresponding pressure points on the feet, hands, ears, scalp, and many other places. Regular stimulation of the pressure points on the feet (or whatever area you feel drawn to work on) can accelerate healing on all levels, any place in the body. Reflexology can also maintain those body points — and the body as a whole — in harmony and balance. Many people feel that if they have problems with one or a few parts of the body, then only those pressure points need to be stimulated. This can actually cause greater imbalance in the body. Certainly, you can pay more attention to those power points where you know extreme problems exist, but it is very important to maintain a regular stimulation of all the points so as to ensure a continuing holistic balance and integration of the entire body. One can have reflexology done alone as a separate therapy, or included as part of a full body massage, Aromatherapy or any other healing modality.

## Reiki

Reiki is a tremendously powerful way of working with body energies to balance and align the body and free blockages, which allows healing on many levels. Unfortunately, one of the organizations that teach this therapy has been very greedy, charging thousands of dollars for multi-levels of training. We highly recommend this form of energy healing and have no qualms about the therapists. We only warn those who choose to be trained in Reiki that you may be brainwashed into believing that you need multi-levels of mastership and thousands of dollars in fees for something that can be genuinely learned and practiced in a very short period of time. Use your intuitive insights and internal guidance to determine if this is for you, and if so, where you will obtain your training. The organization we refer to above does not have monopoly rights on teaching Reiki. You can learn this technique from other sources. There are those who will gladly teach this technique for very reasonable fees.

## Voice Dialogue Therapy

All of us have many different voices inside our heads. Some of these voices are very loving and supportive. Others can be very negative, condemning and destructive. Voice Dialogue Therapy is an opportunity to become as consciously aware as possible of just how many voices we have speaking to us inside our heads, how often the different voices speak, what triggers each voice to begin talking to us, and which voices are the most dominating and controlling.

With this therapy, the person sits in a separate chair for each voice. Sometimes there may only be two or three chairs, while other individuals may end up with ten or twelve or more chairs to sit in. The therapist is very attuned to hear and feel the different voices that start speaking through our voice as he or she asks continuous questions. Each time the therapist senses that a different voice is speaking through our answers, we are directed to a particular chair that is assigned to each voice. We discover in a short period of time how many voices are speaking and which ones are most in control by how often we change chairs, and which chairs we sit in most often.

Examples of the different kinds of voices speaking through us are: the critic, guilt, the over-protective caretaker, anger, fear, sympathy, denial, lack of clarity, grief, negative expectation, the over-analyzer, hope, and the most commonly sat-in chair of all: the avoider ("I don't know").

This is a tremendously powerful therapy to illustrate our self-obstructing and self-destructive patterns so that we can become more aware of where they come from, how often they are triggered, and how we can be more aware of when they are present in our consciousness and speech. That way, we can take responsibility and authority of our lives and more consciously choose how we think, feel and communicate.

# Epilogue

We have presented in the last chapter of this book many different therapies that individuals can seek and experience in order to determine what best supports them in their own healing and self-discovery. We choose not to give you the names and phone numbers of organizations and therapists because (1) this book is not a directory of organizations and therapists which would be a whole book in and of itself and (2) our choice is to provide you with the opportunity to take active responsibility in finding that which will assist you in your healing process.

Too many people look for someone to tell them what to do or more often to simply do it all for them. You learn to develop and trust your own intuition and inner-discernment through day-to-day experience. So long as we hold on to fear of failure or that voice in our minds that says, "I don't know what to do, I don't know where to begin and I don't understand," we sabotage our possibility to experience and develop our own discernment and intuition. Dare to make "mistakes," understanding that in reality there is no such thing as a mistake. Experience is our best teacher. Until we are willing to let ourselves experience and choose on our own, we deny ourselves this opportunity for self-growth, self-honoring and self-love.

The authors of this book, Dr. Marcy Foley Davidsson, William Shaffer and Kent Davidsson, offer among them their experience in Akashic Record readings, dream counseling, training in the use of therapeutic quality essential oils, Health Readings, Naturopathic Care, Past-Life Regression Therapy, DNA reprogramming, Sound Therapy, individualized Vibrational Remedy Programs (including homeopathy, gem elixirs and flower essences), Rebirthing, other books and many seminars dedicated to teaching and supporting individuals in discovering and developing their own spiritual truth and path.

You are welcome to visit our web site or call the Toll Free number and request our catalog of products and services offered. However, we are only three healing facilitators among many. We urge you to go inside and ask to be guided to the most appropriate facilitator for you to work with at any given time. Readers are welcome to share with us your healing challenges and what body symbology you notice, or to offer any comments with us about the material in this book. You may contact us at kornax68@hotmail.com.

For those who are willing to take the initiative in gathering people together for seminars, we the authors are ready to work with you. We look forward to sharing our knowledge and experience with those who truly choose to heal themselves. In the following pages we will now share information about our other books on healing and spiritual development. These books are available through Kornax Enterprises at the Toll Free number listed on the Title Page.

In sharing all of the above with you,

the ball is now in your court!

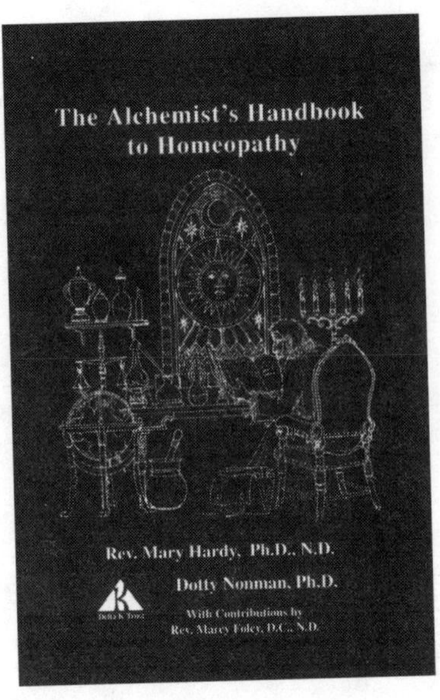
The Alchemist's Handbook
to Homeopathy
Rev. Mary Hardy, Ph.D., N.D.
Dotty Nonman, Ph.D.
With Contributions by
Rev. Marcy Foley, D.C., N.D.

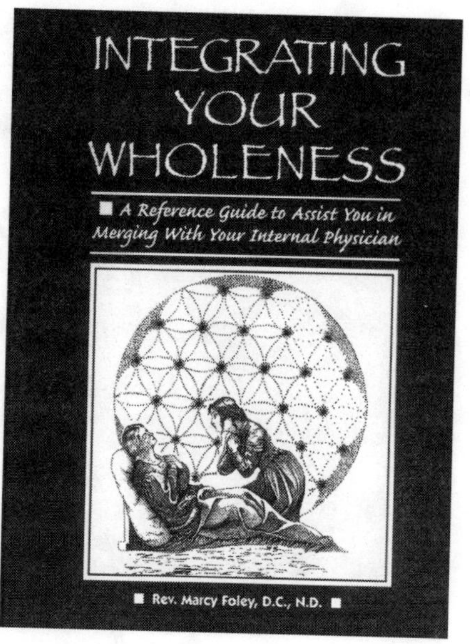


This book is Dr. Foley's professional study of the best in natural healing containing wisdom from the teachings of Rev. Hanna Kroeger, Dr. John Christopher, Dr. Gary Young, and others, interspersed with Dr. Foley's Naturopathic understanding of the healing process. *Integrating Your Wholeness* is a compendium of knowledge and experience in natural healing for the physician or lay person.

Discussed in this book are factors which can contribute to ill health including allergies, poisons, worms and parasites, trauma, congestion, residues and infections. Diet and natural foods cooking ideas are presented. Dr. Foley identifies symptoms of detoxification, understanding a cleansing crises, fasting procedures and contraindications for going on a fast. Dr. Foley addresses writing a vision for your life and the spiritual component of healing as well. 306 pages (8 ½"X 11")

$45 Plus $5 Shipping & Handling

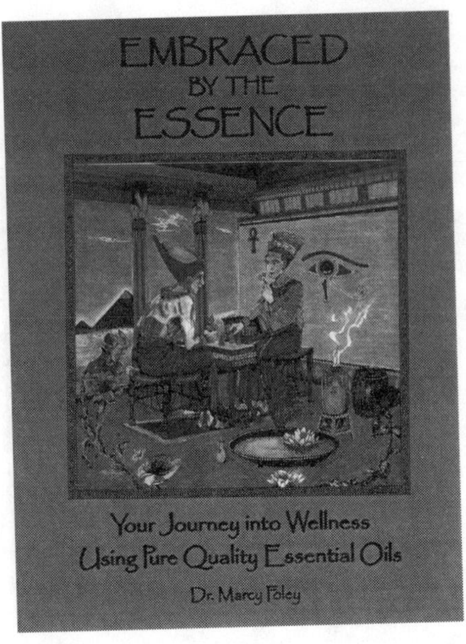


Dr. Foley's most popular book is her reference manual on essential oils. This textbook teaches an introduction on Aromatherapy, essential oil chemistry and the Naturopathic method of healing utilizing humankind's first recorded medicines. Dr. Foley outlines what factors may not be functioning optimally in the body, and various ways to raise the frequency of the vital force in the body, so the body can heal itself.

Included in this book are suggestions of essential oils and related supplements to assist the body in restoring optimal functioning levels. A wonderful part of this book is the chapter on emotional well being. Also included is information on first aid and trauma, degenerative disease, and information for designing your own wellness program. 376 pages 8 1/2" x 11"

$33 Plus $5.50 Shipping & Handling